GOLD'S GYM®

workout journal

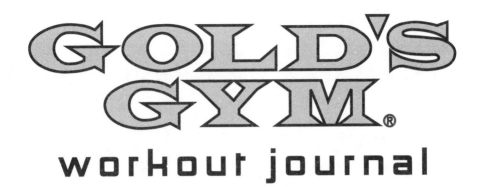

workout journal

Cathy Sassin

CB

CONTEMPORARY BOOKS

Library of Congress Cataloging-in-Publication Data

Sassin, Cathy.
    Gold's Gym workout journal / Cathy Sassin.
        p.   cm.
    ISBN 0-8092-9751-5
    1. Bodybuilding.   2. Weight training.   3. Nutrition.   4. Cardiovascular
fitness.   I. Gold's Gym.   II. Title.
RC1220.W44 S275   2000
613.7—dc21
                                                  00-22697
                                                        CIP

Cover design by Todd Petersen
Front-cover photograph courtesy of Gold's Gym International, Inc.
Back-cover photograph copyright © Jay Farbman
Interior design by Hespenheide Design

Published by Contemporary Books
A division of NTC/Contemporary Publishing Group, Inc.
4255 West Touhy Avenue, Lincolnwood (Chicago), Illinois 60712-1975 U.S.A.
Copyright © 2001 by Gold's Gym Merchandising, Inc.
Printed in the United States of America
International Standard Book Number: 0-8092-9751-5
03 04 05 RRD 18 17 16 15 14 13 12 11 10 9 8 7 6 5 4

CONTENTS

INTRODUCTION

Congratulations on your commitment to fitness! You have chosen Gold's Gym, the leader in fitness, as your guide. Regardless of your fitness level, fitness goals, or fitness history, this exercise and nutrition journal will help you monitor your progress. Keeping a journal not only helps analyze progress, but it's also a great motivator for sticking to your fitness plan.

Here at Gold's Gym, we have worked with thousands of professional athletes, celebrities, models, fitness models, recreational athletes, people with medical concerns and/or dieting histories, and people who simply want to look and feel better. Whether your concern is bodyfat loss; muscle gain; improving speed, strength, or endurance; or simply improving overall health, there are a number of variables that must be considered, each as important as the next. While many of these are individual metabolic variables that will affect your rate of progress—age, gender, body composition, family genetics, nutritional history, exercise history, meal patterns, current type and level of activity, and your commitment level—this journal focuses on the primary three: nutrition, cardiovascular (aerobic) exercise, and weight training.

The Basic Three

Nutrition

The first and most often overlooked key to any fitness goal is
nutrition! How we eat directly affects how the human body stores
fat, releases energy, and counters the effects of aging; put simply,
it determines how much energy we have during the day.

Cardiovascular Exercise

The second crucial element to an effective fitness program is cardiovascular exercise; a type of exercise involving the major muscle
groups, that can be sustained consistently for at least 30 minutes,
at least four times per week. Cardiovascular exercise not only
helps reduce heart disease, blood pressure, cholesterol, effects of
diabetes and other diseases, but also helps dramatically in reducing bodyfat and gaining muscle tissue. The muscle tissue is the
tissue in the body where stored fat is converted into energy, there-
fore the better your cardiovascular condition and the more muscle tissue you have, the more effectively your body will burn fat.

Weight Training

The third component to overall fitness is weight training. For
those interested in increasing athletic performance, making gains
in lean mass (muscle) or changing the shape of their body, proper
weight training application is crucial. For anyone interested in
losing bodyfat only, weight training can be revisited after starting
and maintaining a consistent nutrition and cardiovascular exercise program.

The Total Fitness Triangle

These three elements are the points of the total fitness triangle.
They must all be in balance in order to achieve and maintain any
fitness goal. Each of the three will be briefly discussed in the following three chapters. When you have read and digested that
information, you will be ready to begin keeping your personal
records using the weekly journal pages.

GOLD'S GYM®

workout journal

1

NUTRITION

To achieve any long-term fitness goal, nutrition is the key. The components of nutrition that must be considered, understood, and determined **individually** are discussed in this chapter. In the Appendix at the back of your journal you will find a nutritional breakdown of many foods to help you in designing your own diet.

Caloric Intake
(How Many Calories Do I Need?)

Rather than consider how many calories you need per day, it is more effective to consider how many calories you need in each meal. The human body doesn't start and stop on a 24-hour basis; it is a constantly working machine, using and storing energy all day and night. In order to determine how many calories you need per meal, you will need to have your body composition measured, then use the calculations in Table 1A on page 6 to learn how to break down your meals. When you have finished all the Table 1A calculations, you will be ready to plan your meals using the food content tables in the Appendix.

Your total overall weight is not the complete picture. How much of your weight is metabolically active tissue (bones, joints, ligaments, organs, muscle—the tissue we need to feed with calories to keep functioning) and how much is simply bodyfat (the body's storage containers for extra calories is bodyfat) is more important. The scale doesn't give us this information. Total weight lost or gained is highly misleading. You will need to know how many pounds of fat you're losing and how many pounds of lean tissue (muscle) you're gaining. Measuring body composition is the only way to determine this.

Body composition testing is normally done at universities, at health clubs equipped with a nutrition or trainer's center, and at some chiropractic clinics, or it can be done at home with the use of a manual caliper unit or bio-impedence scale. It is recommended that you have your bodyfat tested by a professional, preferably the same person each time you have a measurement taken. Once you have your body composition measured, you can use Table 1A to help determine some general nutrition guidelines to reach your individual fitness goal.

Meal Frequency
(How Often Should I Eat?)

Just as important as caloric intake per meal is your meal frequency. In order to make forward progress toward any fitness goal, the brain needs adequate fuel. Glucose (simple sugar, the result of carbohydrate breakdown) is the only source of fuel the brain uses. If the brain is low on fuel (glucose), it will warn you. The only way the brain knows that it has adequate fuel levels is by how much glucose is in the bloodstream (measured by blood glucose levels). If the blood sugar levels are low, you will experience one or more symptoms of *hypoglycemia*:

- Headache
- Fatigue, lethargy
- Lack of concentration
- Irritability
- Mood swings
- Lightheadedness, dizziness, shakiness
- Caffeine cravings
- Carbohydrate cravings
- Sugar cravings
- Hunger

Once you experience hypoglycemic symptoms, it's too late: the fuel tank is empty and the brain will already be shifting into fat storage mode. It will be impossible to have strong workouts, to maintain consistent energy levels, or to make forward progress toward any fitness goal while in a hypoglycemic state. Normally, hypoglycemia leads to the carbohydrate binge cycle: the brain eventually forces the hunger drive to cause an overconsumption of (or bingeing on) carbohydrate-rich foods, which leads to a flooding of the hormone insulin into the bloodstream, causing fat stores to increase. This is normally followed by feeling full or guilty, causing a long gap until the next meal. The blood sugar levels fall again during that gap, hypoglycemia is once again prevalent, and the cycle starts over (see Chart 1A).

In order to avoid hypoglycemic symptoms and the carbohydrate binge cycle, it is necessary to eat a meal at least every four hours. The general rule is to eat within an hour of waking and continue to eat every four hours until a couple of hours before bedtime. If your meals are balanced properly, you will feel satisfied after each meal, then be ready for your next meal four hours later.

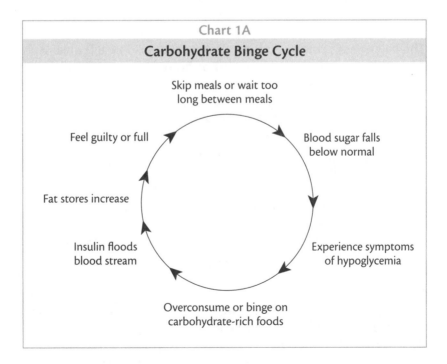

Chart 1A

Carbohydrate Binge Cycle

Skip meals or wait too long between meals

Feel guilty or full

Blood sugar falls below normal

Fat stores increase

Insulin floods blood stream

Experience symptoms of hypoglycemia

Overconsume or binge on carbohydrate-rich foods

This works out to four meals per day, assuming you are getting six to eight hours of sleep most nights. Normally, after you have followed a well-designed nutrition and exercise program for a couple of weeks, your sugar cravings disappear, and it becomes necessary to eat even more frequently, possibly every 3 to 3½ hours.

Examples of Meal Schedules

Wake by	Meal 1	Meal 2	Meal 3	Meal 4	In bed after
5 am	6 am	10 am	2 pm	6 pm	8 pm
6 am	7 am	11 am	3 pm	7 pm	9 pm
7 am	8 am	12 pm	4 pm	8 pm	10 pm
8 am	9 am	1 pm	5 pm	9 pm	11 pm

Nutrient Ratios
(How Much Protein, Carbohydrates, and Fat Should I Eat in Each Meal?)

The balance of proteins, carbohydrates, and fats in each meal is just as critical as caloric intake and meal frequency. These are the *macronutrients* necessary to reach any fitness goal. (The *micronutrients*—vitamins, minerals, and water—will be discussed briefly later in this chapter). Any diet program sent out to the general population will not take individual variables into account. For example, some people, based on their current eating habits, food preferences, activity level, and fitness goals, require more protein in their diet, some more carbohydrates, others more fat. Most people will see initial results with any standard diet program but will have trouble maintaining the diet and the results over time. There is no reason to give up any foods you like for the rest of your life. If you crave a food, it simply means your body is missing something that that particular food provides. For example, if you crave sugar or carbohydrates, your blood sugar level is low. It is not necessary to deprive your body of any nutrient to achieve your goals; for example, you don't have to cut your carbohydrate intake down to 40 percent or less of your current intake to lose bodyfat.

Chart 1B			
The Macronutrients			
Function	**Result**	**Hormonal Response**	**Result**
Carbohydrates Carbohydrates provide energy for all metabolic function, especially the brain and nervous system; they are needed in the diet to burn fat in the cells.	Increase in blood sugar levels. Stimulation of insulin production.	The secretion of insulin accelerates the storage of glucose and fatty acids.	Decrease in blood sugar levels.
Proteins Protein helps in building and repair of all tissues and manufacturing of enzymes and hormones.	Stimulation of glucagon production.	Secretion of glucagon accelerates the breakdown and release of glucose and fatty acids.	Increase in blood sugar levels and inhibition of fat storage.
Fats Fats provide the body with essential fatty acids and are necessary to assimilate fat soluble vitamins.	Promotes the secretion of CCK.	Regulates the secretion rate of bile.	Slows the emptying of the stomach, provides a feeling of fullness and appetite suppression.

Once you have your body composition checked, you can use Table 1A to help you determine your general nutrition guidelines. Chart 1B gives you an outline of the macronutrients, their role in the diet, and the hormonal effects they produce.

It is important to balance the macronutrients in each meal. Ideally, you want just enough carbohydrates in each meal to give the brain the fuel it needs and to supply energy for all metabolic

Table 1A

Calculating Calories per Meal and Nutrient Ratios

1. Have your body composition measured by a professional or check your bodyfat percentage and weight at home with a skin caliper unit or bio-impedance scale.

2. Calculate your lean mass ratio and pounds of fat:

   Weight (____ lb.) × percentage bodyfat (____%) = ____ lb. of fat

   Total weight (____ lb.) − lb. of fat (____ lb.) = lb. lean tissue (____ lb.)

3. Calculate your calories per day based on the following information:

Activity Level	Women	Men
Sedentary (less than 1 hour of exercise per day)	13 calories/lb. lean	14–16 calories/lb. lean
Moderately Active (1 to 2 hours of exercise per day)	14–16 calories/lb. lean	17–19 calories/lb. lean
Highly Active (more than 2 hours of exercise per day)	17–20 calories/lb. lean	20–22 calories/lb. lean

   ____ Calories/lb. lean × ____ lb. lean tissue = ____ calories per day

4. Calculate your calories per meal:

   ____ Calories per day ÷ 4 (to eat every four hours) = ____ calories per meal

   ____ Calories per day ÷ 5 (to eat every three hours) = ____ calories per meal

functions without causing an overproduction of insulin. (Overproduction of insulin will stimulate fat storage through activating the *lipoprotein lipase enzyme system*). If it does not obtain enough carbohydrates for fuel from each meal, the body craves sugar and carbohydrates and exhibits other symptoms of hypoglycemia.

Each meal should also consist of enough protein to support your workouts, rebuild and repair tissue, and cause a release of *glucagon*, a hormone that helps stimulate the release of fat from storage via the hormone sensitive lipoprotein lipase enzyme sys-

---
Table 1A cont.
---

5. Calculate your macronutrient ratios in calories:

   Protein: ___ calories per meal × .25 = ___ calories in protein/meal

   Carbohydrates: ___ calories per meal × .55 = ___ calories in carbohydrates/meal

   Fats: ___ calories per meal × .20 = ___ calories in fat/meal

   - If lean mass gain is your primary goal, multiply your protein by .30 and your carbohydrates by .50.

   - If you currently eat very little protein, start by multiplying your protein by .20; then increase it to .25 gradually over time.

6. Calculate your macronutrient ratios in grams:

   1 gram protein = 4 calories

   1 gram carbohydrates = 4 calories

   1 gram fat = 9 calories

   ___ Calories protein ÷ 4 calories per gram = ___ grams protein/meal

   ___ Calories carbohydrates ÷ 4 calories per gram = ___ grams carbohydrates/meal

   ___ Calories fat ÷ 9 calories per gram = ___ grams fat/ meal

---

tem, but not so much glucagon that it will be taxing on the liver and kidneys or will cause fat storage. It is difficult to achieve any fitness goal without adequate dietary protein.

Each meal should have enough dietary fat to supply your body with the essential fatty acids and to help prolong the emptying time of the stomach without causing fat storage. Too little dietary fat in each meal causes sugar and carbohydrate cravings as well as other symptoms of hypoglycemia due to fluctuating blood sugar levels.

Micronutrients: Vitamins, Minerals, and Water

Vitamins and minerals perform highly specific metabolic functions, especially in energy metabolism. They do not actually provide energy to the body, but they do help release the energy provided by the macronutrients. Vitamin and mineral supplementation is typically recommended to ensure at least the Recommended Daily Allowance (RDA) of all the essential micronutrients in the diet.

The minimum daily intake of water for a sedentary individual is approximately three quarts per day. One gallon (four quarts) per day is ideal for someone who is very active.

2

CARDIOVASCULAR EXERCISE

Consistent cardiovascular exercise is necessary for any health or fitness goal. Cardiovascular exercise dramatically reduces the effects of hypertension, diabetes, high cholesterol, and many other diseases of age. It is also mandatory for reducing bodyfat permanently, increasing lean mass, increasing the metabolic rate and fat-burning enzymes within the muscles, and promoting favorable biochemical and intramuscular changes. Cardiovascular exercise should not be painful, and, like proper nutrition, needs to be determined on an individual basis.

The specific factors used in determining a proper cardiovascular prescription are the type, frequency, duration, and intensity of exercises.

Type
(What Kind of Exercise Should I Do?)

Any exercise that includes the major muscle groups and can be maintained for at least 30 consecutive minutes in each session can be considered beneficial for cardiovascular conditioning. These are aerobic-type exercises requiring consistent oxygen uptake and causing the body to utilize predominantly fat from storage. Examples include walking, hiking, jogging, running, stairmaster, cross trainer, elliptical trainer, nordic ski machine, swimming, aquatic running, cycling, spinning, and some aerobics classes, to name a few.

Activities where your heart rate fluctuates high and low are not considered aerobic cardiovascular exercise. These activities are great for increasing the strength of the heart and are beneficial for overall conditioning, cross training, and fun, but they are not always optimum for burning fat. Examples include tennis, sprinting, some high-intensity aerobics classes, football, kickboxing, volleyball, and weight training, among others.

The best type of aerobic cardiovascular exercise is the type you enjoy and will do. Whether performed at a gym, on a machine at home in front of the television, or outside, it shouldn't feel like a task. Refer to the information under the heading "Intensity" if you feel reluctant to start cardiovascular exercise.

Frequency
(How Often Should I Do Cardio?)

To lose fat and gain lean mass; to improve speed, strength, or endurance; or simply to improve overall health and slow the effects of aging, cardiovascular exercise should be done at least four times per week. Refer to Table 2A to help determine where to start and how to progress toward your individual fitness goal.

Duration
(How Long Should I Exercise?)

Any aerobic exercise done for at least 30 minutes per session will be conducive to all fitness goals. If you are not in the habit of doing any cardiovascular exercise, start with 15–20 minutes for the first week, then increase the duration based on Table 2A.

Intensity
(How Hard Should I Exercise?)

The level of intensity will vary greatly based on your individual fitness goals. If fat loss or muscle gain are the primary goals, you

---

Table 2A

Cardiovascular Prescription

Find a comfortable level for yourself and then gradually work up to higher levels over the weeks with the following schedule:

	Frequency (sessions/week)	Duration (minutes/session)	Intensity (% heart rate)
Start	4	30	60–70
Work up to	4	40	70–75
	5	30	70–75
	4	45	70–75
	5	40	70–75
	4	50	70–75
	5	45	70–75
	4	55	70–75
	5	50	70–75
	6	40	70–75
	4	60	70–75
	5	55	70–75
	6	45	70–75
	4	45	75–80
	5	60	70–75
	6	50	70–75
	4	45	75–80
	5	40	75–80
	6	60	70–75
	5	45	75–80
	6	40	75–80
	5	50	75–80
	6	45	75–80
	5	55	75–80
	6	50	75–80
	5	60	75–80
	6	55	75–80

continued

Table 2A cont.

Frequency (sessions/week)	Duration (minutes/session)	Intensity (% heart rate)
5	45	75–85
6	40	75–85
7	45	70–75
5	50	75–85
6	45	75–85
7	50	70–75
5	55	75–85
6	50	75–85
7	55	70–75
5	60	75–85
6	55	75–85
7	60	70–75
6	60	75–85
7	45	75–85
7	50	75–85
7	55	75–85
7	60	75–85

If you are completely inactive, start with 4 days per week × 15 minutes per session at any comfortable intensity. Check your heart rate every 10 minutes and log your progress in your journal.

will want to exercise at about 70–75% of your maximum effort. This intensity level should be maintained for 30–60 minutes without discomfort. If you aren't in the habit of doing cardiovascular exercise, you can start at 60–70% of your maximum and build up your intensity over the first couple of weeks.

If an increase in speed, strength, or endurance is included in your goals, you will want to exercise at an intensity of 75–85% of your maximum. This intensity is more fatiguing, but you can

---

Table 2B

Calculating Target Heart Rate

1. Calculate maximum heart rate (Max HR):

   220 − your age = _____ beats/minute (Max HR)

2. Calculate your **target heart rate** in beats per minute:

   60%: Max HR (beats/minute) ___ × .60 = ___ beats/minute (target heart rate)

   65%: Max HR (beats/minute) ___ × .65 = ___ beats/minute (target heart rate)

   70%: Max HR (beats/minute) ___ × .70 = ___ beats/minute (target heart rate)

   75%: Max HR (beats/minute) ___ × .75 = ___ beats/minute (target heart rate)

   80%: Max HR (beats/minute) ___ × .80 = ___ beats/minute (target heart rate)

   85%: Max HR (beats/minute) ___ × .85 = ___ beats/minute (target heart rate)

3. Convert your target heart rate to beats per 10 seconds:

   ___ beats per minute ÷ 6 = ___ beats/10 seconds (target heart rate)

Warning: Caffeine, Ma Huang, Ephedrine, and other stimulants will cause an increase in heart rate while exercising.

After following a consistent cardiovascular program, it is normal to feel that you are working harder at the same heart rate over the weeks. Your heart will be in better condition and will beat fewer times per minute to supply the same oxygen demands to the working muscles. You will also feel stronger and have more endurance.

---

work into it by slowly increasing the intensity level as per Table 2A over a few weeks.

The only way to make sure you are exercising efficiently for your goals is by measuring your heart rate. The use of a heart rate monitor is ideal and highly recommended for effective exercise. (Some cardio machines are equipped with a built-in heart-rate monitor). You can also measure your heart rate by checking your pulse every 10 minutes during exercise. This method is a little less accurate due to the slight drop in your heart rate when you stop to check, but it is better to check frequently than to continue a cardio program that may be ineffective for your goal. Many people exercise, but don't see the results they expect because the exercise is inefficient for their goal, leading to frustration. (Refer to Table 2B to learn how to calculate your target heart rate).

To check your pulse, stop exercising momentarily, place your index and middle fingers gently against your radial artery (on the thumb side of your wrist), your carotid artery (in the groove on one side of your throat just where the chin meets the neck), or your temporal artery (at your temple). Once you locate your pulse, count the number of beats in 10 seconds. Continue to exercise, then check again every 10 minutes to make sure you stay at the proper intensity level. Refer to Table 2A to help you design your own cardiovascular program.

3

WEIGHT TRAINING

The third crucial element to your fitness plan is proper weight training. The benefits of weight training, aside from increasing muscle size, include increase in muscle, bone, connective tissue, and tendon strength; increase in muscular endurance, intramuscular fuel stores, neurological reaction time, mental concentration, and power; and an overall feeling of well-being.

There are different weight training methods for different goals. In order to increase size and strength, it is not necessary to "lift as much weight as possible," but rather to maximize the force-generating capacity of the muscle being worked through perfect application. When any given muscle is required to generate more force than it is used to, it will adapt by becoming bigger and/or stronger. Proper biomechanics are necessary to maximize the impact of the muscle being worked, reduce the recruitment of auxiliary muscle groups, and reduce the risk of injury. Training specifically for your goals requires focus, intensity, consistency, and commitment.

To train for an increase in size and/or strength, a *split body-part workout routine* is best. To train for overall strength, change in shape, or sports specificity, *an upper body/lower body split routine* can be used. If you are just starting a weight training program, it is best to have a professional trainer show you how to perform proper weight training application. A full-body *circuit training* routine works well to adapt all the muscles to resistance training, to avoid excessive soreness, and to reduce the risk of injury. Refer to Table 3A for sample weight training routines.

Locate the weight training schedule that best fits your goals, using the examples provided in Table 3A. Choose different exercises for each muscle group based on the equipment you have available, and follow the set and rep schemes provided. It is always best to seek the guidance of a professional trainer in order to maximize the effectiveness of your workouts and avoid the risk of injury.

Be sure to include cardiovascular workouts in your overall training design.

Table 3A

Sample Weight Training Schedules

For Increasing Size and Strength

Regular Training Schedule	Body Parts/ Session	Exercises/ Body Part	Sets/ Exercise	Well-executed Reps/Set	Rest Intervals Between Sets
2 days on, 1 day off	1 major, 2 minor muscle groups	2–3	3–4	4–8	60–90 seconds

---

BODYBUILDER SPLIT ROUTINE

Rotate the exercises in each workout so that each time you train a muscle group, you use different exercises from Table 3B for the muscle group you are training. This will help constantly stimulate growth.

SAMPLE REGULAR TRAINING SCHEDULE

Day 1: Chest, Triceps, Abdominals

Day 2: Back, Biceps, Forearms

Day 3: off

Day 4: Quadriceps, Hamstrings, Calves

Day 5: Shoulders, Lower Back, Abdominals

Day 6: off

Day 7: Chest, Triceps, Abdominals

Day 8: Back, Biceps, Forearms

Day 9: off

Day 10: Quadriceps, Hamstrings, Calves

Day 11: Shoulders, Lower Back, Abdominals

Day 12: off

Keep cycling muscle groups around according to this "2 days on, 1 day off" training schedule regardless of the day of the week.

continued

Table 3A cont.

Overall Strength/Sports Specificity

Weekly Training Schedule	Body Parts/ Session	Exercises/ Body Part	Sets/ Exercise	Well-executed Reps/Set	Rest Intervals Between Sets
2 days on, 1 day off	Upper body/ lower body split	3	3–4	10–20	60 seconds
2 days on, 2 days off					

UPPER BODY/LOWER BODY SPLIT ROUTINE

Rotate the exercises in each workout so that each time you train a muscle group, you use different exercises from Table 3B for that muscle group.

SAMPLE WEEKLY TRAINING SCHEDULE

Day 1: Chest, Shoulders, Biceps, Triceps, Abdominals

Day 2: Quadriceps, Hamstrings, Calves, Back

Day 3: off

Day 4: Chest, Shoulders, Biceps, Triceps, Abdominals

Day 5: Quadriceps, Hamstrings, Calves, Back

Day 6: off

Day 7: off

Day 8: Chest, Shoulders, Biceps, Triceps, Abdominals

Day 9: Quadriceps, Hamstrings, Calves, Back

Day 10: off

Keep cycling muscle groups on the "2 days on, 1 day off, 2 days on, 2 days off" training schedule, regardless of the day of the week.

Table 3A cont.

For Full-Body Workout

Weekly Training Schedule	Body Parts/ Session	Exercises/ Body Part	Sets/ Exercise	Well-executed Reps/Set	Rest Intervals Between Sets
1–3 sessions/ week	Full-body workout	1	2	15–25	30 seconds

CIRCUIT TRAINING ROUTINE

Rotate the exercise for each muscle group once every four workouts.

SAMPLE WEEKLY TRAINING SCHEDULE

Day 1: Quadriceps, Hamstrings, Calves, Shoulders, Back, Chest, Biceps, Triceps, Forearms, Abdominals

Day 2: off

Day 3: Quadriceps, Hamstrings, Calves, Shoulders, Back, Chest, Biceps, Triceps, Forearms, Abdominals

Day 4: off

Day 5: Quadriceps, Hamstrings, Calves, Shoulders, Back, Chest, Biceps, Triceps, Forearms, Abdominals

Day 6: off

Day 7: off

Day 8: Quadriceps, Hamstrings, Calves, Shoulders, Back, Chest, Biceps, Triceps, Forearms, Abdominals

Day 9: off

Day 10: Quadriceps, Hamstrings, Calves, Shoulders, Back, Chest, Biceps, Triceps, Forearms, Abdominals

Day 11: off

Day 12: Quadriceps, Hamstrings, Calves, Shoulders, Back, Chest, Biceps, Triceps, Forearms, Abdominals

Table 3B

Weight Training Exercise Selections

PECTORALS (CHEST)

Barbell Bench Press

Dumbbell Bench Press

Smith Machine Bench Press

Barbell Incline Press

Dumbbell Incline Bench Press

Smith Machine Incline Bench Press

Flat Dumbbell Flyes

Incline Dumbbell Flyes

Machine Seated Press

Cable Crossovers

Dumbbell Pullovers

Machine Pec Deck

Machine Flyes

Parallel Dips

LATISSIMUS DORSI (BACK)

Close-Grip Chin-Ups

Wide-Grip Pull-Downs

Close-Grip Pull-Downs

Seated Cable Rows

Reverse-Grip Seated Cable Rows

Reverse-Grip Pull-Downs

Smith Machine Bent-Over Rows

One-Arm Dumbbell Pulls

Hyperextensions (lower back)

Partial Deadlifts (lower back)

DELTOIDS (SHOULDERS)

Seated Smith Machine Press

Seated Dumbbell Press

Seated Behind-the-Neck Smith Machine Press

Seated Machine Press

Wide-Grip Upright Rows

Close-Grip Upright Rows

Seated Dumbbell Side Laterals

Seated Bent-Over Dumbbell Laterals

Standing Alternate Dumbbell Front Laterals

TRAPEZIUS (TRAPS)

Dumbbell Shrugs

Posterior Barbell Shrugs

BICEPS BRACHII (BICEPS)

Standing Barbell Curls

Seated Alternate Dumbbell Curls

Seated Incline Dumbbell Curls

Preacher Curls

Standing Alternate Dumbbell Curls

Alternate Dumbbell Preacher Curls

Standing Cable Curls

Table 3B cont.

Weight Training Exercise Selections

BICEPS BRACHIALIS (BICEPS)

Seated Hammer Dumbbell Curls

Reverse-Grip Preacher Curls

Standing Reverse-Grip Barbell Curls

TRICEPS BRACHII (TRICEPS)

Triceps Cable Pressdown

Reverse-Grip Triceps Cable Pressdown

Lying Triceps Extensions

Lying Dumbbell Hammer Extensions

Seated Overhead Dumbbell Extensions

Close-Grip Cable Pressdowns

Close-Grip Bench Press

Hammer-Grip Triceps Cable Extensions

Hammer-Grip Overhead Cable
Extensions

Dumbbell Kickbacks

Seated One-Arm Dumbbell Extensions

Seated Overhead Cable Extensions

QUADRICEPS (THIGHS)

Seated Leg Extensions

Angled Leg Press

Duck Hack Squats

Smith Machine Front Squats

Smith Machine Back Squats

Vertical Leg Press

Horizontal Leg Press

Seated Cable Thigh Flyes

HAMSTRINGS

Lying Leg Curls

Standing Alternate Leg Curls

Barbell Stiff-Legged Deadlifts

GASTROCNEMIUS (UPPER CALVES)

Angled Toe Press

Vertical Toe Press

SOLEUS (LOWER CALVES)

Donkey Calf Raise

Seated Calf Raise

Standing Calf Raise

Angled Calf Raise

ABDOMINALS

Angled Sit-Ups

Lying Leg Raises

Wall Crunches

Hanging Knee Tucks

Decline Crunches

Decline Leg Raises

Alternate Knee Tucks

4

WORKOUT
JOURNAL

Regardless of your ultimate fitness goal, maintaining a sound and consistent nutrition and exercise program is the key to your success. Gold's Gym is proud to help you log your progress. In addition to completing the journal pages each day, record your progress each week on the chart that follows.

There are more resources available from the mecca of body-building; they can be found on our website: www.goldsgym.com. We wish you the best of luck in reaching all your short- and long-term fitness goals!

Weekly Body Composition Progress Chart

Start	Date	Weight	% Bodyfat	Pounds Lean	Pounds Fat
Week 1					
Week 2					
Week 3					
Week 4					
Week 5					
Week 6					
Week 7					
Week 8					
Week 9					
Week 10					
Week 11					
Week 12					

Nutrition Journal

DATE _____   WEEK _____   DAY _____

Meal Time	Meal	Foods	Total Calories	Grams Protein	Grams Carbs	Grams Fat	Meal Comments
_____ am/pm	1						
			_____ total	_____ total	_____ total	_____ total	
_____ am/pm	2						
			_____ total	_____ total	_____ total	_____ total	
_____ am/pm	3						
			_____ total	_____ total	_____ total	_____ total	
_____ am/pm	4						
			_____ total	_____ total	_____ total	_____ total	
_____ am/pm	5						
			_____ total	_____ total	_____ total	_____ total	

Exercise Journal

Weight Training

REPETITION SCHEME _____   REST INTERVALS _____
DATE _____   TIME _____   PRE-WORKOUT ENERGY LEVEL _____

Muscle Group	Exercise	Warm-up	Set 1	Set 2	Set 3	Set 4

Cardiovascular Exercise

Type	Total Cardio Time	Time in HR Range	Heart Rate
Bike			
Treadmill			
Stairclimber			
Run			
Aerobics class			
Other			

Nutrition Journal

DATE _____   WEEK _____   DAY _____

Meal Time	Meal	Foods	Total Calories	Grams Protein	Grams Carbs	Grams Fat	Meal Comments
_____ am/pm	1						
			_____ total	_____ total	_____ total	_____ total	
_____ am/pm	2						
			_____ total	_____ total	_____ total	_____ total	
_____ am/pm	3						
			_____ total	_____ total	_____ total	_____ total	
_____ am/pm	4						
			_____ total	_____ total	_____ total	_____ total	
_____ am/pm	5						
			_____ total	_____ total	_____ total	_____ total	

Exercise Journal

Weight Training

REPETITION SCHEME _____   REST INTERVALS _____

DATE _____   TIME _____   PRE-WORKOUT ENERGY LEVEL _____

Muscle Group	Exercise	Warm-up	Set 1	Set 2	Set 3	Set 4

Cardiovascular Exercise

Type	Total Cardio Time	Time in HR Range	Heart Rate
Bike			
Treadmill			
Stairclimber			
Run			
Aerobics class			
Other			

Nutrition Journal

DATE _____   WEEK _____   DAY _____

Meal Time	Meal	Foods	Total Calories	Grams Protein	Grams Carbs	Grams Fat	Meal Comments
_____ am/pm	1						
			total	total	total	total	
_____ am/pm	2						
			total	total	total	total	
_____ am/pm	3						
			total	total	total	total	
_____ am/pm	4						
			total	total	total	total	
_____ am/pm	5						
			total	total	total	total	

Exercise Journal

Weight Training

REPETITION SCHEME _____   REST INTERVALS _____
DATE _____   TIME _____   PRE-WORKOUT ENERGY LEVEL _____

Muscle Group	Exercise	Warm-up	Set 1	Set 2	Set 3	Set 4

Cardiovascular Exercise

Type	Total Cardio Time	Time in HR Range	Heart Rate
Bike			
Treadmill			
Stairclimber			
Run			
Aerobics class			
Other			

Nutrition Journal

DATE _____   WEEK _____   DAY _____

Meal Time	Meal	Foods	Total Calories	Grams Protein	Grams Carbs	Grams Fat	Meal Comments
_____ am/pm	1						
			_____ total	_____ total	_____ total	_____ total	
_____ am/pm	2						
			_____ total	_____ total	_____ total	_____ total	
_____ am/pm	3						
			_____ total	_____ total	_____ total	_____ total	
_____ am/pm	4						
			_____ total	_____ total	_____ total	_____ total	
_____ am/pm	5						
			_____ total	_____ total	_____ total	_____ total	

Exercise Journal

Weight Training

REPETITION SCHEME _____   REST INTERVALS _____
DATE _____   TIME _____   PRE-WORKOUT ENERGY LEVEL _____

Muscle Group	Exercise	Warm-up	Set 1	Set 2	Set 3	Set 4

Cardiovascular Exercise

Type	Total Cardio Time	Time in HR Range	Heart Rate
Bike			
Treadmill			
Stairclimber			
Run			
Aerobics class			
Other			

Nutrition Journal

DATE _____   WEEK _____   DAY _____

Meal Time	Meal	Foods	Total Calories	Grams Protein	Grams Carbs	Grams Fat	Meal Comments
_____ am/pm	1						
			___ total	___ total	___ total	___ total	
_____ am/pm	2						
			___ total	___ total	___ total	___ total	
_____ am/pm	3						
			___ total	___ total	___ total	___ total	
_____ am/pm	4						
			___ total	___ total	___ total	___ total	
_____ am/pm	5						
			___ total	___ total	___ total	___ total	

Exercise Journal

Weight Training

REPETITION SCHEME _____   REST INTERVALS _____
DATE _____   TIME _____   PRE-WORKOUT ENERGY LEVEL _____

Muscle Group	Exercise	Warm-up	Set 1	Set 2	Set 3	Set 4

Cardiovascular Exercise

Type	Total Cardio Time	Time in HR Range	Heart Rate
Bike			
Treadmill			
Stairclimber			
Run			
Aerobics class			
Other			

Nutrition Journal

DATE _____   WEEK _____   DAY _____

Meal Time	Meal	Foods	Total Calories	Grams Protein	Grams Carbs	Grams Fat	Meal Comments
_____ am/pm	1						
			_____ total	_____ total	_____ total	_____ total	
_____ am/pm	2						
			_____ total	_____ total	_____ total	_____ total	
_____ am/pm	3						
			_____ total	_____ total	_____ total	_____ total	
_____ am/pm	4						
			_____ total	_____ total	_____ total	_____ total	
_____ am/pm	5						
			_____ total	_____ total	_____ total	_____ total	

Exercise Journal

Weight Training

REPETITION SCHEME _____   REST INTERVALS _____
DATE _____   TIME _____   PRE-WORKOUT ENERGY LEVEL _____

Muscle Group	Exercise	Warm-up	Set 1	Set 2	Set 3	Set 4

Cardiovascular Exercise

Type	Total Cardio Time	Time in HR Range	Heart Rate
Bike			
Treadmill			
Stairclimber			
Run			
Aerobics class			
Other			

Nutrition Journal

DATE _____   WEEK _____   DAY _____

Meal Time	Meal	Foods	Total Calories	Grams Protein	Grams Carbs	Grams Fat	Meal Comments
_____ am/pm	1						
			total	total	total	total	
_____ am/pm	2						
			total	total	total	total	
_____ am/pm	3						
			total	total	total	total	
_____ am/pm	4						
			total	total	total	total	
_____ am/pm	5						
			total	total	total	total	

Exercise Journal

Weight Training

REPETITION SCHEME _____   REST INTERVALS _____
DATE _____   TIME _____   PRE-WORKOUT ENERGY LEVEL _____

Muscle Group	Exercise	Warm-up	Set 1	Set 2	Set 3	Set 4

Cardiovascular Exercise

Type	Total Cardio Time	Time in HR Range	Heart Rate
Bike			
Treadmill			
Stairclimber			
Run			
Aerobics class			
Other			

Nutrition Journal

DATE _____   WEEK _____   DAY _____

Meal Time	Meal	Foods	Total Calories	Grams Protein	Grams Carbs	Grams Fat	Meal Comments
_____ am/pm	1						
			_____ total	_____ total	_____ total	_____ total	
_____ am/pm	2						
			_____ total	_____ total	_____ total	_____ total	
_____ am/pm	3						
			_____ total	_____ total	_____ total	_____ total	
_____ am/pm	4						
			_____ total	_____ total	_____ total	_____ total	
_____ am/pm	5						
			_____ total	_____ total	_____ total	_____ total	

Exercise Journal

Weight Training

REPETITION SCHEME _____   REST INTERVALS _____
DATE _____   TIME _____   PRE-WORKOUT ENERGY LEVEL _____

Muscle Group	Exercise	Warm-up	Set 1	Set 2	Set 3	Set 4

Cardiovascular Exercise

Type	Total Cardio Time	Time in HR Range	Heart Rate
Bike			
Treadmill			
Stairclimber			
Run			
Aerobics class			
Other			

Nutrition Journal

DATE _____   WEEK _____   DAY _____

Meal Time	Meal	Foods	Total Calories	Grams Protein	Grams Carbs	Grams Fat	Meal Comments
_____ am/pm	1						
			_____ total	_____ total	_____ total	_____ total	
_____ am/pm	2						
			_____ total	_____ total	_____ total	_____ total	
_____ am/pm	3						
			_____ total	_____ total	_____ total	_____ total	
_____ am/pm	4						
			_____ total	_____ total	_____ total	_____ total	
_____ am/pm	5						
			_____ total	_____ total	_____ total	_____ total	

Exercise Journal

Weight Training

REPETITION SCHEME _____   REST INTERVALS _____
DATE _____   TIME _____   PRE-WORKOUT ENERGY LEVEL _____

Muscle Group	Exercise	Warm-up	Set 1	Set 2	Set 3	Set 4

Cardiovascular Exercise

Type	Total Cardio Time	Time in HR Range	Heart Rate
Bike			
Treadmill			
Stairclimber			
Run			
Aerobics class			
Other			

Nutrition Journal

DATE _____   WEEK _____   DAY _____

Meal Time	Meal	Foods	Total Calories	Grams Protein	Grams Carbs	Grams Fat	Meal Comments
_____ am/pm	1						
			_____ total	_____ total	_____ total	_____ total	
_____ am/pm	2						
			_____ total	_____ total	_____ total	_____ total	
_____ am/pm	3						
			_____ total	_____ total	_____ total	_____ total	
_____ am/pm	4						
			_____ total	_____ total	_____ total	_____ total	
_____ am/pm	5						
			_____ total	_____ total	_____ total	_____ total	

Exercise Journal

Weight Training

REPETITION SCHEME _____ REST INTERVALS _____
DATE _____ TIME _____ PRE-WORKOUT ENERGY LEVEL _____

Muscle Group	Exercise	Warm-up	Set 1	Set 2	Set 3	Set 4

Cardiovascular Exercise

Type	Total Cardio Time	Time in HR Range	Heart Rate
Bike			
Treadmill			
Stairclimber			
Run			
Aerobics class			
Other			

Nutrition Journal

DATE _____   WEEK _____   DAY _____

Meal Time	Meal	Foods	Total Calories	Grams Protein	Grams Carbs	Grams Fat	Meal Comments
_____ am/pm	1						
			_____ total	_____ total	_____ total	_____ total	
_____ am/pm	2						
			_____ total	_____ total	_____ total	_____ total	
_____ am/pm	3						
			_____ total	_____ total	_____ total	_____ total	
_____ am/pm	4						
			_____ total	_____ total	_____ total	_____ total	
_____ am/pm	5						
			_____ total	_____ total	_____ total	_____ total	

Exercise Journal

Weight Training

REPETITION SCHEME _____   REST INTERVALS _____
DATE _____   TIME _____   PRE-WORKOUT ENERGY LEVEL _____

Muscle Group	Exercise	Warm-up	Set 1	Set 2	Set 3	Set 4

Cardiovascular Exercise

Type	Total Cardio Time	Time in HR Range	Heart Rate
Bike			
Treadmill			
Stairclimber			
Run			
Aerobics class			
Other			

Nutrition Journal

DATE _____   WEEK _____   DAY _____

Meal Time	Meal	Foods	Total Calories	Grams Protein	Grams Carbs	Grams Fat	Meal Comments
_____ am/pm	1		_____ total	_____ total	_____ total	_____ total	
_____ am/pm	2		_____ total	_____ total	_____ total	_____ total	
_____ am/pm	3		_____ total	_____ total	_____ total	_____ total	
_____ am/pm	4		_____ total	_____ total	_____ total	_____ total	
_____ am/pm	5		_____ total	_____ total	_____ total	_____ total	

Exercise Journal

Weight Training

REPETITION SCHEME _____   REST INTERVALS _____
DATE _____   TIME _____   PRE-WORKOUT ENERGY LEVEL _____

Muscle Group	Exercise	Warm-up	Set 1	Set 2	Set 3	Set 4

Cardiovascular Exercise

Type	Total Cardio Time	Time in HR Range	Heart Rate
Bike			
Treadmill			
Stairclimber			
Run			
Aerobics class			
Other			

Nutrition Journal

DATE _____   WEEK _____   DAY _____

Meal Time	Meal	Foods	Total Calories	Grams Protein	Grams Carbs	Grams Fat	Meal Comments
_____ am/pm	1						
			_____ total	_____ total	_____ total	_____ total	
_____ am/pm	2						
			_____ total	_____ total	_____ total	_____ total	
_____ am/pm	3						
			_____ total	_____ total	_____ total	_____ total	
_____ am/pm	4						
			_____ total	_____ total	_____ total	_____ total	
_____ am/pm	5						
			_____ total	_____ total	_____ total	_____ total	

Exercise Journal

Weight Training

REPETITION SCHEME _____   REST INTERVALS _____
DATE _____   TIME _____   PRE-WORKOUT ENERGY LEVEL _____

Muscle Group	Exercise	Warm-up	Set 1	Set 2	Set 3	Set 4

Cardiovascular Exercise

Type	Total Cardio Time	Time in HR Range	Heart Rate
Bike			
Treadmill			
Stairclimber			
Run			
Aerobics class			
Other			

Nutrition Journal

DATE _____   WEEK _____   DAY _____

Meal Time	Meal	Foods	Total Calories	Grams Protein	Grams Carbs	Grams Fat	Meal Comments
_____ am/pm	1						
			_____ total	_____ total	_____ total	_____ total	
_____ am/pm	2						
			_____ total	_____ total	_____ total	_____ total	
_____ am/pm	3						
			_____ total	_____ total	_____ total	_____ total	
_____ am/pm	4						
			_____ total	_____ total	_____ total	_____ total	
_____ am/pm	5						
			_____ total	_____ total	_____ total	_____ total	

Exercise Journal

Weight Training

REPETITION SCHEME _____   REST INTERVALS _____
DATE _____   TIME _____   PRE-WORKOUT ENERGY LEVEL _____

Muscle Group	Exercise	Warm-up	Set 1	Set 2	Set 3	Set 4

Cardiovascular Exercise

Type	Total Cardio Time	Time in HR Range	Heart Rate
Bike			
Treadmill			
Stairclimber			
Run			
Aerobics class			
Other			

Nutrition Journal

DATE _____   WEEK _____   DAY _____

Meal Time	Meal	Foods	Total Calories	Grams Protein	Grams Carbs	Grams Fat	Meal Comments
_____ am/pm	1						
			___ total	___ total	___ total	___ total	
_____ am/pm	2						
			___ total	___ total	___ total	___ total	
_____ am/pm	3						
			___ total	___ total	___ total	___ total	
_____ am/pm	4						
			___ total	___ total	___ total	___ total	
_____ am/pm	5						
			___ total	___ total	___ total	___ total	

Exercise Journal

Weight Training

REPETITION SCHEME _____   REST INTERVALS _____
DATE _____   TIME _____   PRE-WORKOUT ENERGY LEVEL _____

Muscle Group	Exercise	Warm-up	Set 1	Set 2	Set 3	Set 4

Cardiovascular Exercise

Type	Total Cardio Time	Time in HR Range	Heart Rate
Bike			
Treadmill			
Stairclimber			
Run			
Aerobics class			
Other			

Nutrition Journal

DATE _____   WEEK _____   DAY _____

Meal Time	Meal	Foods	Total Calories	Grams Protein	Grams Carbs	Grams Fat	Meal Comments
_____ am/pm	1						
			_____ total	_____ total	_____ total	_____ total	
_____ am/pm	2						
			_____ total	_____ total	_____ total	_____ total	
_____ am/pm	3						
			_____ total	_____ total	_____ total	_____ total	
_____ am/pm	4						
			_____ total	_____ total	_____ total	_____ total	
_____ am/pm	5						
			_____ total	_____ total	_____ total	_____ total	

Exercise Journal

Weight Training

REPETITION SCHEME _____ REST INTERVALS _____

DATE _____ TIME _____ PRE-WORKOUT ENERGY LEVEL _____

Muscle Group	Exercise	Warm-up	Set 1	Set 2	Set 3	Set 4

Cardiovascular Exercise

Type	Total Cardio Time	Time in HR Range	Heart Rate
Bike			
Treadmill			
Stairclimber			
Run			
Aerobics class			
Other			

Nutrition Journal

DATE _____   WEEK _____   DAY _____

Meal Time	Meal	Foods	Total Calories	Grams Protein	Grams Carbs	Grams Fat	Meal Comments
_____ am/pm	1						
			_____ total	_____ total	_____ total	_____ total	
_____ am/pm	2						
			_____ total	_____ total	_____ total	_____ total	
_____ am/pm	3						
			_____ total	_____ total	_____ total	_____ total	
_____ am/pm	4						
			_____ total	_____ total	_____ total	_____ total	
_____ am/pm	5						
			_____ total	_____ total	_____ total	_____ total	

Exercise Journal

Weight Training

REPETITION SCHEME _____   REST INTERVALS _____
DATE _____   TIME _____   PRE-WORKOUT ENERGY LEVEL _____

Muscle Group	Exercise	Warm-up	Set 1	Set 2	Set 3	Set 4

Cardiovascular Exercise

Type	Total Cardio Time	Time in HR Range	Heart Rate
Bike			
Treadmill			
Stairclimber			
Run			
Aerobics class			
Other			

Nutrition Journal

DATE _____   WEEK _____   DAY _____

Meal Time	Meal	Foods	Total Calories	Grams Protein	Grams Carbs	Grams Fat	Meal Comments
_____ am/pm	1						
			_____ total	_____ total	_____ total	_____ total	
_____ am/pm	2						
			_____ total	_____ total	_____ total	_____ total	
_____ am/pm	3						
			_____ total	_____ total	_____ total	_____ total	
_____ am/pm	4						
			_____ total	_____ total	_____ total	_____ total	
_____ am/pm	5						
			_____ total	_____ total	_____ total	_____ total	

Exercise Journal

Weight Training

REPETITION SCHEME _____   REST INTERVALS _____
DATE _____   TIME _____   PRE-WORKOUT ENERGY LEVEL _____

Muscle Group	Exercise	Warm-up	Set 1	Set 2	Set 3	Set 4

Cardiovascular Exercise

Type	Total Cardio Time	Time in HR Range	Heart Rate
Bike			
Treadmill			
Stairclimber			
Run			
Aerobics class			
Other			

Nutrition Journal

DATE _____   WEEK _____   DAY _____

Meal Time	Meal	Foods	Total Calories	Grams Protein	Grams Carbs	Grams Fat	Meal Comments
_____ am/pm	1						
			_____ total	_____ total	_____ total	_____ total	
_____ am/pm	2						
			_____ total	_____ total	_____ total	_____ total	
_____ am/pm	3						
			_____ total	_____ total	_____ total	_____ total	
_____ am/pm	4						
			_____ total	_____ total	_____ total	_____ total	
_____ am/pm	5						
			_____ total	_____ total	_____ total	_____ total	

Exercise Journal

Weight Training

REPETITION SCHEME _____   REST INTERVALS _____
DATE _____   TIME _____   PRE-WORKOUT ENERGY LEVEL _____

Muscle Group	Exercise	Warm-up	Set 1	Set 2	Set 3	Set 4

Cardiovascular Exercise

Type	Total Cardio Time	Time in HR Range	Heart Rate
Bike			
Treadmill			
Stairclimber			
Run			
Aerobics class			
Other			

Nutrition Journal

DATE _____   WEEK _____   DAY _____

Meal Time	Meal	Foods	Total Calories	Grams Protein	Grams Carbs	Grams Fat	Meal Comments
_____ am/pm	1						
			_____ total	_____ total	_____ total	_____ total	
_____ am/pm	2						
			_____ total	_____ total	_____ total	_____ total	
_____ am/pm	3						
			_____ total	_____ total	_____ total	_____ total	
_____ am/pm	4						
			_____ total	_____ total	_____ total	_____ total	
_____ am/pm	5						
			_____ total	_____ total	_____ total	_____ total	

Exercise Journal

Weight Training

REPETITION SCHEME _____   REST INTERVALS _____
DATE _____   TIME _____   PRE-WORKOUT ENERGY LEVEL _____

Muscle Group	Exercise	Warm-up	Set 1	Set 2	Set 3	Set 4

Cardiovascular Exercise

Type	Total Cardio Time	Time in HR Range	Heart Rate
Bike			
Treadmill			
Stairclimber			
Run			
Aerobics class			
Other			

Nutrition Journal

DATE _____   WEEK _____   DAY _____

Meal Time	Meal	Foods	Total Calories	Grams Protein	Grams Carbs	Grams Fat	Meal Comments
_____ am/pm	1						
			_____ total	_____ total	_____ total	_____ total	
_____ am/pm	2						
			_____ total	_____ total	_____ total	_____ total	
_____ am/pm	3						
			_____ total	_____ total	_____ total	_____ total	
_____ am/pm	4						
			_____ total	_____ total	_____ total	_____ total	
_____ am/pm	5						
			_____ total	_____ total	_____ total	_____ total	

Exercise Journal

Weight Training

REPETITION SCHEME _____   REST INTERVALS _____
DATE _____   TIME _____   PRE-WORKOUT ENERGY LEVEL _____

Muscle Group	Exercise	Warm-up	Set 1	Set 2	Set 3	Set 4

Cardiovascular Exercise

Type	Total Cardio Time	Time in HR Range	Heart Rate
Bike			
Treadmill			
Stairclimber			
Run			
Aerobics class			
Other			

Nutrition Journal

DATE _____   WEEK _____   DAY _____

Meal Time	Meal	Foods	Total Calories	Grams Protein	Grams Carbs	Grams Fat	Meal Comments
_____ am/pm	1						
			_____ total	_____ total	_____ total	_____ total	
_____ am/pm	2						
			_____ total	_____ total	_____ total	_____ total	
_____ am/pm	3						
			_____ total	_____ total	_____ total	_____ total	
_____ am/pm	4						
			_____ total	_____ total	_____ total	_____ total	
_____ am/pm	5						
			_____ total	_____ total	_____ total	_____ total	

Exercise Journal

Weight Training

REPETITION SCHEME _____   REST INTERVALS _____
DATE _____   TIME _____   PRE-WORKOUT ENERGY LEVEL _____

Muscle Group	Exercise	Warm-up	Set 1	Set 2	Set 3	Set 4

Cardiovascular Exercise

Type	Total Cardio Time	Time in HR Range	Heart Rate
Bike			
Treadmill			
Stairclimber			
Run			
Aerobics class			
Other			

Nutrition Journal

DATE _____   WEEK _____   DAY _____

Meal Time	Meal	Foods	Total Calories	Grams Protein	Grams Carbs	Grams Fat	Meal Comments
_____ am/pm	1		_____ total	_____ total	_____ total	_____ total	
_____ am/pm	2		_____ total	_____ total	_____ total	_____ total	
_____ am/pm	3		_____ total	_____ total	_____ total	_____ total	
_____ am/pm	4		_____ total	_____ total	_____ total	_____ total	
_____ am/pm	5		_____ total	_____ total	_____ total	_____ total	

Exercise Journal

Weight Training

REPETITION SCHEME _____   REST INTERVALS _____
DATE _____   TIME _____   PRE-WORKOUT ENERGY LEVEL _____

Muscle Group	Exercise	Warm-up	Set 1	Set 2	Set 3	Set 4

Cardiovascular Exercise

Type	Total Cardio Time	Time in HR Range	Heart Rate
Bike			
Treadmill			
Stairclimber			
Run			
Aerobics class			
Other			

Nutrition Journal

DATE _____   WEEK _____   DAY _____

Meal Time	Meal	Foods	Total Calories	Grams Protein	Grams Carbs	Grams Fat	Meal Comments
_____ am/pm	1						
			_____ total	_____ total	_____ total	_____ total	
_____ am/pm	2						
			_____ total	_____ total	_____ total	_____ total	
_____ am/pm	3						
			_____ total	_____ total	_____ total	_____ total	
_____ am/pm	4						
			_____ total	_____ total	_____ total	_____ total	
_____ am/pm	5						
			_____ total	_____ total	_____ total	_____ total	

Exercise Journal

Weight Training

REPETITION SCHEME _____   REST INTERVALS _____
DATE _____   TIME _____   PRE-WORKOUT ENERGY LEVEL _____

Muscle Group	Exercise	Warm-up	Set 1	Set 2	Set 3	Set 4

Cardiovascular Exercise

Type	Total Cardio Time	Time in HR Range	Heart Rate
Bike			
Treadmill			
Stairclimber			
Run			
Aerobics class			
Other			

Nutrition Journal

DATE _____   WEEK _____   DAY _____

Meal Time	Meal	Foods	Total Calories	Grams Protein	Grams Carbs	Grams Fat	Meal Comments
_____ am/pm	1						
			___ total	___ total	___ total	___ total	
_____ am/pm	2						
			___ total	___ total	___ total	___ total	
_____ am/pm	3						
			___ total	___ total	___ total	___ total	
_____ am/pm	4						
			___ total	___ total	___ total	___ total	
_____ am/pm	5						
			___ total	___ total	___ total	___ total	

Exercise Journal

Weight Training

REPETITION SCHEME _____   REST INTERVALS _____
DATE _____   TIME _____   PRE-WORKOUT ENERGY LEVEL _____

Muscle Group	Exercise	Warm-up	Set 1	Set 2	Set 3	Set 4

Cardiovascular Exercise

Type	Total Cardio Time	Time in HR Range	Heart Rate
Bike			
Treadmill			
Stairclimber			
Run			
Aerobics class			
Other			

Nutrition Journal

DATE _____   WEEK _____   DAY _____

Meal Time	Meal	Foods	Total Calories	Grams Protein	Grams Carbs	Grams Fat	Meal Comments
_____ am/pm	1						
			_____ total	_____ total	_____ total	_____ total	
_____ am/pm	2						
			_____ total	_____ total	_____ total	_____ total	
_____ am/pm	3						
			_____ total	_____ total	_____ total	_____ total	
_____ am/pm	4						
			_____ total	_____ total	_____ total	_____ total	
_____ am/pm	5						
			_____ total	_____ total	_____ total	_____ total	

Exercise Journal

Weight Training

REPETITION SCHEME _____   REST INTERVALS _____
DATE _____   TIME _____   PRE-WORKOUT ENERGY LEVEL _____

Muscle Group	Exercise	Warm-up	Set 1	Set 2	Set 3	Set 4

Cardiovascular Exercise

Type	Total Cardio Time	Time in HR Range	Heart Rate
Bike			
Treadmill			
Stairclimber			
Run			
Aerobics class			
Other			

Nutrition Journal

DATE _____   WEEK _____   DAY _____

Meal Time	Meal	Foods	Total Calories	Grams Protein	Grams Carbs	Grams Fat	Meal Comments
_____ am/pm	1						
			___ total	___ total	___ total	___ total	
_____ am/pm	2						
			___ total	___ total	___ total	___ total	
_____ am/pm	3						
			___ total	___ total	___ total	___ total	
_____ am/pm	4						
			___ total	___ total	___ total	___ total	
_____ am/pm	5						
			___ total	___ total	___ total	___ total	

Exercise Journal

Weight Training

REPETITION SCHEME _____   REST INTERVALS _____
DATE _____   TIME _____   PRE-WORKOUT ENERGY LEVEL _____

Muscle Group	Exercise	Warm-up	Set 1	Set 2	Set 3	Set 4

Cardiovascular Exercise

Type	Total Cardio Time	Time in HR Range	Heart Rate
Bike			
Treadmill			
Stairclimber			
Run			
Aerobics class			
Other			

Nutrition Journal

DATE _____   WEEK _____   DAY _____

Meal Time	Meal	Foods	Total Calories	Grams Protein	Grams Carbs	Grams Fat	Meal Comments
_____ am/pm	1						
			_____ total	_____ total	_____ total	_____ total	
_____ am/pm	2						
			_____ total	_____ total	_____ total	_____ total	
_____ am/pm	3						
			_____ total	_____ total	_____ total	_____ total	
_____ am/pm	4						
			_____ total	_____ total	_____ total	_____ total	
_____ am/pm	5						
			_____ total	_____ total	_____ total	_____ total	

Exercise Journal

Weight Training

REPETITION SCHEME _____   REST INTERVALS _____

DATE _____   TIME _____   PRE-WORKOUT ENERGY LEVEL _____

Muscle Group	Exercise	Warm-up	Set 1	Set 2	Set 3	Set 4

Cardiovascular Exercise

Type	Total Cardio Time	Time in HR Range	Heart Rate
Bike			
Treadmill			
Stairclimber			
Run			
Aerobics class			
Other			

Nutrition Journal

DATE _____   WEEK _____   DAY _____

Meal Time	Meal	Foods	Total Calories	Grams Protein	Grams Carbs	Grams Fat	Meal Comments
_____ am/pm	1						
			_____ total	_____ total	_____ total	_____ total	
_____ am/pm	2						
			_____ total	_____ total	_____ total	_____ total	
_____ am/pm	3						
			_____ total	_____ total	_____ total	_____ total	
_____ am/pm	4						
			_____ total	_____ total	_____ total	_____ total	
_____ am/pm	5						
			_____ total	_____ total	_____ total	_____ total	

Exercise Journal

Weight Training

REPETITION SCHEME _____   REST INTERVALS _____
DATE _____   TIME _____   PRE-WORKOUT ENERGY LEVEL _____

Muscle Group	Exercise	Warm-up	Set 1	Set 2	Set 3	Set 4

Cardiovascular Exercise

Type	Total Cardio Time	Time in HR Range	Heart Rate
Bike			
Treadmill			
Stairclimber			
Run			
Aerobics class			
Other			

Nutrition Journal

DATE _____   WEEK _____   DAY _____

Meal Time	Meal	Foods	Total Calories	Grams Protein	Grams Carbs	Grams Fat	Meal Comments
_____ am/pm	1						
			_____ total	_____ total	_____ total	_____ total	
_____ am/pm	2						
			_____ total	_____ total	_____ total	_____ total	
_____ am/pm	3						
			_____ total	_____ total	_____ total	_____ total	
_____ am/pm	4						
			_____ total	_____ total	_____ total	_____ total	
_____ am/pm	5						
			_____ total	_____ total	_____ total	_____ total	

Exercise Journal

Weight Training

REPETITION SCHEME _____   REST INTERVALS _____
DATE _____   TIME _____   PRE-WORKOUT ENERGY LEVEL _____

Muscle Group	Exercise	Warm-up	Set 1	Set 2	Set 3	Set 4

Cardiovascular Exercise

Type	Total Cardio Time	Time in HR Range	Heart Rate
Bike			
Treadmill			
Stairclimber			
Run			
Aerobics class			
Other			

Nutrition Journal

DATE _____   WEEK _____   DAY _____

Meal Time	Meal	Foods	Total Calories	Grams Protein	Grams Carbs	Grams Fat	Meal Comments
_____ am/pm	1						
			total	total	total	total	
_____ am/pm	2						
			total	total	total	total	
_____ am/pm	3						
			total	total	total	total	
_____ am/pm	4						
			total	total	total	total	
_____ am/pm	5						
			total	total	total	total	

Exercise Journal

Weight Training

REPETITION SCHEME _____   REST INTERVALS _____
DATE _____   TIME _____   PRE-WORKOUT ENERGY LEVEL _____

Muscle Group	Exercise	Warm-up	Set 1	Set 2	Set 3	Set 4

Cardiovascular Exercise

Type	Total Cardio Time	Time in HR Range	Heart Rate
Bike			
Treadmill			
Stairclimber			
Run			
Aerobics class			
Other			

Nutrition Journal

DATE _____   WEEK _____   DAY _____

Meal Time	Meal	Foods	Total Calories	Grams Protein	Grams Carbs	Grams Fat	Meal Comments
_____ am/pm	1						
			_____ total	_____ total	_____ total	_____ total	
_____ am/pm	2						
			_____ total	_____ total	_____ total	_____ total	
_____ am/pm	3						
			_____ total	_____ total	_____ total	_____ total	
_____ am/pm	4						
			_____ total	_____ total	_____ total	_____ total	
_____ am/pm	5						
			_____ total	_____ total	_____ total	_____ total	

Exercise Journal

Weight Training

REPETITION SCHEME _____   REST INTERVALS _____
DATE _____   TIME _____   PRE-WORKOUT ENERGY LEVEL _____

Muscle Group	Exercise	Warm-up	Set 1	Set 2	Set 3	Set 4

Cardiovascular Exercise

Type	Total Cardio Time	Time in HR Range	Heart Rate
Bike			
Treadmill			
Stairclimber			
Run			
Aerobics class			
Other			

Nutrition Journal

DATE _____   WEEK _____   DAY _____

Meal Time	Meal	Foods	Total Calories	Grams Protein	Grams Carbs	Grams Fat	Meal Comments
_____ am/pm	1						
			_____ total	_____ total	_____ total	_____ total	
_____ am/pm	2						
			_____ total	_____ total	_____ total	_____ total	
_____ am/pm	3						
			_____ total	_____ total	_____ total	_____ total	
_____ am/pm	4						
			_____ total	_____ total	_____ total	_____ total	
_____ am/pm	5						
			_____ total	_____ total	_____ total	_____ total	

Exercise Journal

Weight Training

REPETITION SCHEME _____   REST INTERVALS _____
DATE _____   TIME _____   PRE-WORKOUT ENERGY LEVEL _____

Muscle Group	Exercise	Warm-up	Set 1	Set 2	Set 3	Set 4

Cardiovascular Exercise

Type	Total Cardio Time	Time in HR Range	Heart Rate
Bike			
Treadmill			
Stairclimber			
Run			
Aerobics class			
Other			

Nutrition Journal

DATE _____   WEEK _____   DAY _____

Meal Time	Meal	Foods	Total Calories	Grams Protein	Grams Carbs	Grams Fat	Meal Comments
_____ am/pm	1						
			___ total	___ total	___ total	___ total	
_____ am/pm	2						
			___ total	___ total	___ total	___ total	
_____ am/pm	3						
			___ total	___ total	___ total	___ total	
_____ am/pm	4						
			___ total	___ total	___ total	___ total	
_____ am/pm	5						
			___ total	___ total	___ total	___ total	

Exercise Journal

Weight Training

REPETITION SCHEME _____   REST INTERVALS _____
DATE _____   TIME _____   PRE-WORKOUT ENERGY LEVEL _____

Muscle Group	Exercise	Warm-up	Set 1	Set 2	Set 3	Set 4

Cardiovascular Exercise

Type	Total Cardio Time	Time in HR Range	Heart Rate
Bike			
Treadmill			
Stairclimber			
Run			
Aerobics class			
Other			

Nutrition Journal

DATE _____   WEEK _____   DAY _____

Meal Time	Meal	Foods	Total Calories	Grams Protein	Grams Carbs	Grams Fat	Meal Comments
_____ am/pm	1						
			total	total	total	total	
_____ am/pm	2						
			total	total	total	total	
_____ am/pm	3						
			total	total	total	total	
_____ am/pm	4						
			total	total	total	total	
_____ am/pm	5						
			total	total	total	total	

Exercise Journal

Weight Training

REPETITION SCHEME _____   REST INTERVALS _____
DATE _____   TIME _____   PRE-WORKOUT ENERGY LEVEL _____

Muscle Group	Exercise	Warm-up	Set 1	Set 2	Set 3	Set 4

Cardiovascular Exercise

Type	Total Cardio Time	Time in HR Range	Heart Rate
Bike			
Treadmill			
Stairclimber			
Run			
Aerobics class			
Other			

Nutrition Journal

DATE _____   WEEK _____   DAY _____

Meal Time	Meal	Foods	Total Calories	Grams Protein	Grams Carbs	Grams Fat	Meal Comments
_____ am/pm	1						
			total	total	total	total	
_____ am/pm	2						
			total	total	total	total	
_____ am/pm	3						
			total	total	total	total	
_____ am/pm	4						
			total	total	total	total	
_____ am/pm	5						
			total	total	total	total	

Exercise Journal

Weight Training

REPETITION SCHEME _____ REST INTERVALS _____
DATE _____ TIME _____ PRE-WORKOUT ENERGY LEVEL _____

Muscle Group	Exercise	Warm-up	Set 1	Set 2	Set 3	Set 4

Cardiovascular Exercise

Type	Total Cardio Time	Time in HR Range	Heart Rate
Bike			
Treadmill			
Stairclimber			
Run			
Aerobics class			
Other			

Nutrition Journal

DATE _____　　WEEK _____　　DAY _____

Meal Time	Meal	Foods	Total Calories	Grams Protein	Grams Carbs	Grams Fat	Meal Comments
_____ am/pm	1						
			_____ total	_____ total	_____ total	_____ total	
_____ am/pm	2						
			_____ total	_____ total	_____ total	_____ total	
_____ am/pm	3						
			_____ total	_____ total	_____ total	_____ total	
_____ am/pm	4						
			_____ total	_____ total	_____ total	_____ total	
_____ am/pm	5						
			_____ total	_____ total	_____ total	_____ total	

Exercise Journal

Weight Training

REPETITION SCHEME _____   REST INTERVALS _____
DATE _____   TIME _____   PRE-WORKOUT ENERGY LEVEL _____

Muscle Group	Exercise	Warm-up	Set 1	Set 2	Set 3	Set 4

Cardiovascular Exercise

Type	Total Cardio Time	Time in HR Range	Heart Rate
Bike			
Treadmill			
Stairclimber			
Run			
Aerobics class			
Other			

Nutrition Journal

DATE _____   WEEK _____   DAY _____

Meal Time	Meal	Foods	Total Calories	Grams Protein	Grams Carbs	Grams Fat	Meal Comments
_____ am/pm	1						
			_____ total	_____ total	_____ total	_____ total	
_____ am/pm	2						
			_____ total	_____ total	_____ total	_____ total	
_____ am/pm	3						
			_____ total	_____ total	_____ total	_____ total	
_____ am/pm	4						
			_____ total	_____ total	_____ total	_____ total	
_____ am/pm	5						
			_____ total	_____ total	_____ total	_____ total	

Exercise Journal

Weight Training

REPETITION SCHEME _____   REST INTERVALS _____
DATE _____   TIME _____   PRE-WORKOUT ENERGY LEVEL _____

Muscle Group	Exercise	Warm-up	Set 1	Set 2	Set 3	Set 4

Cardiovascular Exercise

Type	Total Cardio Time	Time in HR Range	Heart Rate
Bike			
Treadmill			
Stairclimber			
Run			
Aerobics class			
Other			

Nutrition Journal

DATE _____   WEEK _____   DAY _____

Meal Time	Meal	Foods	Total Calories	Grams Protein	Grams Carbs	Grams Fat	Meal Comments
_____ am/pm	1						
			_____ total	_____ total	_____ total	_____ total	
_____ am/pm	2						
			_____ total	_____ total	_____ total	_____ total	
_____ am/pm	3						
			_____ total	_____ total	_____ total	_____ total	
_____ am/pm	4						
			_____ total	_____ total	_____ total	_____ total	
_____ am/pm	5						
			_____ total	_____ total	_____ total	_____ total	

Exercise Journal

Weight Training

REPETITION SCHEME _____   REST INTERVALS _____
DATE _____   TIME _____   PRE-WORKOUT ENERGY LEVEL _____

Muscle Group	Exercise	Warm-up	Set 1	Set 2	Set 3	Set 4

Cardiovascular Exercise

Type	Total Cardio Time	Time in HR Range	Heart Rate
Bike			
Treadmill			
Stairclimber			
Run			
Aerobics class			
Other			

Nutrition Journal

DATE _____   WEEK _____   DAY _____

Meal Time	Meal	Foods	Total Calories	Grams Protein	Grams Carbs	Grams Fat	Meal Comments
_____ am/pm	1						
			_____ total	_____ total	_____ total	_____ total	
_____ am/pm	2						
			_____ total	_____ total	_____ total	_____ total	
_____ am/pm	3						
			_____ total	_____ total	_____ total	_____ total	
_____ am/pm	4						
			_____ total	_____ total	_____ total	_____ total	
_____ am/pm	5						
			_____ total	_____ total	_____ total	_____ total	

Exercise Journal

Weight Training

REPETITION SCHEME _____   REST INTERVALS _____
DATE _____   TIME _____   PRE-WORKOUT ENERGY LEVEL _____

Muscle Group	Exercise	Warm-up	Set 1	Set 2	Set 3	Set 4

Cardiovascular Exercise

Type	Total Cardio Time	Time in HR Range	Heart Rate
Bike			
Treadmill			
Stairclimber			
Run			
Aerobics class			
Other			

Nutrition Journal

DATE _____   WEEK _____   DAY _____

Meal Time	Meal	Foods	Total Calories	Grams Protein	Grams Carbs	Grams Fat	Meal Comments
_____ am/pm	1						
			_____ total	_____ total	_____ total	_____ total	
_____ am/pm	2						
			_____ total	_____ total	_____ total	_____ total	
_____ am/pm	3						
			_____ total	_____ total	_____ total	_____ total	
_____ am/pm	4						
			_____ total	_____ total	_____ total	_____ total	
_____ am/pm	5						
			_____ total	_____ total	_____ total	_____ total	

Exercise Journal

Weight Training

REPETITION SCHEME _____   REST INTERVALS _____
DATE _____   TIME _____   PRE-WORKOUT ENERGY LEVEL _____

Muscle Group	Exercise	Warm-up	Set 1	Set 2	Set 3	Set 4

Cardiovascular Exercise

Type	Total Cardio Time	Time in HR Range	Heart Rate
Bike			
Treadmill			
Stairclimber			
Run			
Aerobics class			
Other			

Nutrition Journal

DATE _____   WEEK _____   DAY _____

Meal Time	Meal	Foods	Total Calories	Grams Protein	Grams Carbs	Grams Fat	Meal Comments
_____ am/pm	1		_____ total	_____ total	_____ total	_____ total	
_____ am/pm	2		_____ total	_____ total	_____ total	_____ total	
_____ am/pm	3		_____ total	_____ total	_____ total	_____ total	
_____ am/pm	4		_____ total	_____ total	_____ total	_____ total	
_____ am/pm	5		_____ total	_____ total	_____ total	_____ total	

Exercise Journal

Weight Training

REPETITION SCHEME _____   REST INTERVALS _____
DATE _____   TIME _____   PRE-WORKOUT ENERGY LEVEL _____

Muscle Group	Exercise	Warm-up	Set 1	Set 2	Set 3	Set 4

Cardiovascular Exercise

Type	Total Cardio Time	Time in HR Range	Heart Rate
Bike			
Treadmill			
Stairclimber			
Run			
Aerobics class			
Other			

Nutrition Journal

DATE _____   WEEK _____   DAY _____

Meal Time	Meal	Foods	Total Calories	Grams Protein	Grams Carbs	Grams Fat	Meal Comments
_____ am/pm	1						
			total	total	total	total	
_____ am/pm	2						
			total	total	total	total	
_____ am/pm	3						
			total	total	total	total	
_____ am/pm	4						
			total	total	total	total	
_____ am/pm	5						
			total	total	total	total	

Exercise Journal

Weight Training

REPETITION SCHEME _____   REST INTERVALS _____
DATE _____   TIME _____   PRE-WORKOUT ENERGY LEVEL _____

Muscle Group	Exercise	Warm-up	Set 1	Set 2	Set 3	Set 4

Cardiovascular Exercise

Type	Total Cardio Time	Time in HR Range	Heart Rate
Bike			
Treadmill			
Stairclimber			
Run			
Aerobics class			
Other			

Nutrition Journal

DATE _____   WEEK _____   DAY _____

Meal Time	Meal	Foods	Total Calories	Grams Protein	Grams Carbs	Grams Fat	Meal Comments
_____ am/pm	1						
			_____ total	_____ total	_____ total	_____ total	
_____ am/pm	2						
			_____ total	_____ total	_____ total	_____ total	
_____ am/pm	3						
			_____ total	_____ total	_____ total	_____ total	
_____ am/pm	4						
			_____ total	_____ total	_____ total	_____ total	
_____ am/pm	5						
			_____ total	_____ total	_____ total	_____ total	

Exercise Journal

Weight Training

REPETITION SCHEME _____   REST INTERVALS _____
DATE _____   TIME _____   PRE-WORKOUT ENERGY LEVEL _____

Muscle Group	Exercise	Warm-up	Set 1	Set 2	Set 3	Set 4

Cardiovascular Exercise

Type	Total Cardio Time	Time in HR Range	Heart Rate
Bike			
Treadmill			
Stairclimber			
Run			
Aerobics class			
Other			

Nutrition Journal

DATE _____   WEEK _____   DAY _____

Meal Time	Meal	Foods	Total Calories	Grams Protein	Grams Carbs	Grams Fat	Meal Comments
_____ am/pm	1						
			___ total	___ total	___ total	___ total	
_____ am/pm	2						
			___ total	___ total	___ total	___ total	
_____ am/pm	3						
			___ total	___ total	___ total	___ total	
_____ am/pm	4						
			___ total	___ total	___ total	___ total	
_____ am/pm	5						
			___ total	___ total	___ total	___ total	

Exercise Journal

Weight Training

REPETITION SCHEME _____   REST INTERVALS _____
DATE _____   TIME _____   PRE-WORKOUT ENERGY LEVEL _____

Muscle Group	Exercise	Warm-up	Set 1	Set 2	Set 3	Set 4

Cardiovascular Exercise

Type	Total Cardio Time	Time in HR Range	Heart Rate
Bike			
Treadmill			
Stairclimber			
Run			
Aerobics class			
Other			

Nutrition Journal

DATE _____   WEEK _____   DAY _____

Meal Time	Meal	Foods	Total Calories	Grams Protein	Grams Carbs	Grams Fat	Meal Comments
_____ am/pm	1						
			___ total	___ total	___ total	___ total	
_____ am/pm	2						
			___ total	___ total	___ total	___ total	
_____ am/pm	3						
			___ total	___ total	___ total	___ total	
_____ am/pm	4						
			___ total	___ total	___ total	___ total	
_____ am/pm	5						
			___ total	___ total	___ total	___ total	

Exercise Journal

Weight Training

REPETITION SCHEME _____   REST INTERVALS _____

DATE _____   TIME _____   PRE-WORKOUT ENERGY LEVEL _____

Muscle Group	Exercise	Warm-up	Set 1	Set 2	Set 3	Set 4

Cardiovascular Exercise

Type	Total Cardio Time	Time in HR Range	Heart Rate
Bike			
Treadmill			
Stairclimber			
Run			
Aerobics class			
Other			

Nutrition Journal

DATE _____   WEEK _____   DAY _____

Meal Time	Meal	Foods	Total Calories	Grams Protein	Grams Carbs	Grams Fat	Meal Comments
_____ am/pm	1						
			total	total	total	total	
_____ am/pm	2						
			total	total	total	total	
_____ am/pm	3						
			total	total	total	total	
_____ am/pm	4						
			total	total	total	total	
_____ am/pm	5						
			total	total	total	total	

Exercise Journal

Weight Training

REPETITION SCHEME _____   REST INTERVALS _____
DATE _____   TIME _____   PRE-WORKOUT ENERGY LEVEL _____

Muscle Group	Exercise	Warm-up	Set 1	Set 2	Set 3	Set 4

Cardiovascular Exercise

Type	Total Cardio Time	Time in HR Range	Heart Rate
Bike			
Treadmill			
Stairclimber			
Run			
Aerobics class			
Other			

Nutrition Journal

DATE _____   WEEK _____   DAY _____

Meal Time	Meal	Foods	Total Calories	Grams Protein	Grams Carbs	Grams Fat	Meal Comments
_____ am/pm	1						
			_____ total	_____ total	_____ total	_____ total	
_____ am/pm	2						
			_____ total	_____ total	_____ total	_____ total	
_____ am/pm	3						
			_____ total	_____ total	_____ total	_____ total	
_____ am/pm	4						
			_____ total	_____ total	_____ total	_____ total	
_____ am/pm	5						
			_____ total	_____ total	_____ total	_____ total	

Exercise Journal

Weight Training

REPETITION SCHEME _____   REST INTERVALS _____
DATE _____   TIME _____   PRE-WORKOUT ENERGY LEVEL _____

Muscle Group	Exercise	Warm-up	Set 1	Set 2	Set 3	Set 4

Cardiovascular Exercise

Type	Total Cardio Time	Time in HR Range	Heart Rate
Bike			
Treadmill			
Stairclimber			
Run			
Aerobics class			
Other			

Nutrition Journal

DATE _____   WEEK _____   DAY _____

Meal Time	Meal	Foods	Total Calories	Grams Protein	Grams Carbs	Grams Fat	Meal Comments
_____ am/pm	1						
			_____ total	_____ total	_____ total	_____ total	
_____ am/pm	2						
			_____ total	_____ total	_____ total	_____ total	
_____ am/pm	3						
			_____ total	_____ total	_____ total	_____ total	
_____ am/pm	4						
			_____ total	_____ total	_____ total	_____ total	
_____ am/pm	5						
			_____ total	_____ total	_____ total	_____ total	

Exercise Journal

Weight Training

REPETITION SCHEME _____   REST INTERVALS _____
DATE _____   TIME _____   PRE-WORKOUT ENERGY LEVEL _____

Muscle Group	Exercise	Warm-up	Set 1	Set 2	Set 3	Set 4

Cardiovascular Exercise

Type	Total Cardio Time	Time in HR Range	Heart Rate
Bike			
Treadmill			
Stairclimber			
Run			
Aerobics class			
Other			

Nutrition Journal

DATE _____   WEEK _____   DAY _____

Meal Time	Meal	Foods	Total Calories	Grams Protein	Grams Carbs	Grams Fat	Meal Comments
_____ am/pm	1						
			_____ total	_____ total	_____ total	_____ total	
_____ am/pm	2						
			_____ total	_____ total	_____ total	_____ total	
_____ am/pm	3						
			_____ total	_____ total	_____ total	_____ total	
_____ am/pm	4						
			_____ total	_____ total	_____ total	_____ total	
_____ am/pm	5						
			_____ total	_____ total	_____ total	_____ total	

Exercise Journal

Weight Training

REPETITION SCHEME _____   REST INTERVALS _____
DATE _____   TIME _____   PRE-WORKOUT ENERGY LEVEL _____

Muscle Group	Exercise	Warm-up	Set 1	Set 2	Set 3	Set 4

Cardiovascular Exercise

Type	Total Cardio Time	Time in HR Range	Heart Rate
Bike			
Treadmill			
Stairclimber			
Run			
Aerobics class			
Other			

Nutrition Journal

DATE _____   WEEK _____   DAY _____

Meal Time	Meal	Foods	Total Calories	Grams Protein	Grams Carbs	Grams Fat	Meal Comments
_____ am/pm	1						
			_____ total	_____ total	_____ total	_____ total	
_____ am/pm	2						
			_____ total	_____ total	_____ total	_____ total	
_____ am/pm	3						
			_____ total	_____ total	_____ total	_____ total	
_____ am/pm	4						
			_____ total	_____ total	_____ total	_____ total	
_____ am/pm	5						
			_____ total	_____ total	_____ total	_____ total	

Exercise Journal

Weight Training

REPETITION SCHEME _____   REST INTERVALS _____
DATE _____   TIME _____   PRE-WORKOUT ENERGY LEVEL _____

Muscle Group	Exercise	Warm-up	Set 1	Set 2	Set 3	Set 4

Cardiovascular Exercise

Type	Total Cardio Time	Time in HR Range	Heart Rate
Bike			
Treadmill			
Stairclimber			
Run			
Aerobics class			
Other			

Nutrition Journal

DATE _____   WEEK _____   DAY _____

Meal Time	Meal	Foods	Total Calories	Grams Protein	Grams Carbs	Grams Fat	Meal Comments
_____ am/pm	1		___ total	___ total	___ total	___ total	
_____ am/pm	2		___ total	___ total	___ total	___ total	
_____ am/pm	3		___ total	___ total	___ total	___ total	
_____ am/pm	4		___ total	___ total	___ total	___ total	
_____ am/pm	5		___ total	___ total	___ total	___ total	

Exercise Journal

Weight Training

REPETITION SCHEME _____   REST INTERVALS _____
DATE _____   TIME _____   PRE-WORKOUT ENERGY LEVEL _____

Muscle Group	Exercise	Warm-up	Set 1	Set 2	Set 3	Set 4

Cardiovascular Exercise

Type	Total Cardio Time	Time in HR Range	Heart Rate
Bike			
Treadmill			
Stairclimber			
Run			
Aerobics class			
Other			

Nutrition Journal

DATE _____   WEEK _____   DAY _____

Meal Time	Meal	Foods	Total Calories	Grams Protein	Grams Carbs	Grams Fat	Meal Comments
_____ am/pm	1						
			_____ total	_____ total	_____ total	_____ total	
_____ am/pm	2						
			_____ total	_____ total	_____ total	_____ total	
_____ am/pm	3						
			_____ total	_____ total	_____ total	_____ total	
_____ am/pm	4						
			_____ total	_____ total	_____ total	_____ total	
_____ am/pm	5						
			_____ total	_____ total	_____ total	_____ total	

Exercise Journal

Weight Training

REPETITION SCHEME _____   REST INTERVALS _____
DATE _____   TIME _____   PRE-WORKOUT ENERGY LEVEL _____

Muscle Group	Exercise	Warm-up	Set 1	Set 2	Set 3	Set 4

Cardiovascular Exercise

Type	Total Cardio Time	Time in HR Range	Heart Rate
Bike			
Treadmill			
Stairclimber			
Run			
Aerobics class			
Other			

Nutrition Journal

DATE _____   WEEK _____   DAY _____

Meal Time	Meal	Foods	Total Calories	Grams Protein	Grams Carbs	Grams Fat	Meal Comments
_____ am/pm	1						
			_____ total	_____ total	_____ total	_____ total	
_____ am/pm	2						
			_____ total	_____ total	_____ total	_____ total	
_____ am/pm	3						
			_____ total	_____ total	_____ total	_____ total	
_____ am/pm	4						
			_____ total	_____ total	_____ total	_____ total	
_____ am/pm	5						
			_____ total	_____ total	_____ total	_____ total	

Exercise Journal

Weight Training

REPETITION SCHEME _____   REST INTERVALS _____
DATE _____   TIME _____   PRE-WORKOUT ENERGY LEVEL _____

Muscle Group	Exercise	Warm-up	Set 1	Set 2	Set 3	Set 4

Cardiovascular Exercise

Type	Total Cardio Time	Time in HR Range	Heart Rate
Bike			
Treadmill			
Stairclimber			
Run			
Aerobics class			
Other			

Nutrition Journal

DATE _____   WEEK _____   DAY _____

Meal Time	Meal	Foods	Total Calories	Grams Protein	Grams Carbs	Grams Fat	Meal Comments
_____ am/pm	1						
			_____ total	_____ total	_____ total	_____ total	
_____ am/pm	2						
			_____ total	_____ total	_____ total	_____ total	
_____ am/pm	3						
			_____ total	_____ total	_____ total	_____ total	
_____ am/pm	4						
			_____ total	_____ total	_____ total	_____ total	
_____ am/pm	5						
			_____ total	_____ total	_____ total	_____ total	

Exercise Journal

Weight Training

REPETITION SCHEME _____   REST INTERVALS _____
DATE _____   TIME _____   PRE-WORKOUT ENERGY LEVEL _____

Muscle Group	Exercise	Warm-up	Set 1	Set 2	Set 3	Set 4

Cardiovascular Exercise

Type	Total Cardio Time	Time in HR Range	Heart Rate
Bike			
Treadmill			
Stairclimber			
Run			
Aerobics class			
Other			

Nutrition Journal

DATE _____   WEEK _____   DAY _____

Meal Time	Meal	Foods	Total Calories	Grams Protein	Grams Carbs	Grams Fat	Meal Comments
_____ am/pm	1						
			_____ total	_____ total	_____ total	_____ total	
_____ am/pm	2						
			_____ total	_____ total	_____ total	_____ total	
_____ am/pm	3						
			_____ total	_____ total	_____ total	_____ total	
_____ am/pm	4						
			_____ total	_____ total	_____ total	_____ total	
_____ am/pm	5						
			_____ total	_____ total	_____ total	_____ total	

Exercise Journal

Weight Training

REPETITION SCHEME _____   REST INTERVALS _____
DATE _____   TIME _____   PRE-WORKOUT ENERGY LEVEL _____

Muscle Group	Exercise	Warm-up	Set 1	Set 2	Set 3	Set 4

Cardiovascular Exercise

Type	Total Cardio Time	Time in HR Range	Heart Rate
Bike			
Treadmill			
Stairclimber			
Run			
Aerobics class			
Other			

Nutrition Journal

DATE _____   WEEK _____   DAY _____

Meal Time	Meal	Foods	Total Calories	Grams Protein	Grams Carbs	Grams Fat	Meal Comments
_____ am/pm	1						
			_____ total	_____ total	_____ total	_____ total	
_____ am/pm	2						
			_____ total	_____ total	_____ total	_____ total	
_____ am/pm	3						
			_____ total	_____ total	_____ total	_____ total	
_____ am/pm	4						
			_____ total	_____ total	_____ total	_____ total	
_____ am/pm	5						
			_____ total	_____ total	_____ total	_____ total	

Exercise Journal

Weight Training

REPETITION SCHEME _____   REST INTERVALS _____

DATE _____   TIME _____   PRE-WORKOUT ENERGY LEVEL _____

Muscle Group	Exercise	Warm-up	Set 1	Set 2	Set 3	Set 4

Cardiovascular Exercise

Type	Total Cardio Time	Time in HR Range	Heart Rate
Bike			
Treadmill			
Stairclimber			
Run			
Aerobics class			
Other			

Nutrition Journal

DATE _____   WEEK _____   DAY _____

Meal Time	Meal	Foods	Total Calories	Grams Protein	Grams Carbs	Grams Fat	Meal Comments
_____ am/pm	1						
			_____ total	_____ total	_____ total	_____ total	
_____ am/pm	2						
			_____ total	_____ total	_____ total	_____ total	
_____ am/pm	3						
			_____ total	_____ total	_____ total	_____ total	
_____ am/pm	4						
			_____ total	_____ total	_____ total	_____ total	
_____ am/pm	5						
			_____ total	_____ total	_____ total	_____ total	

Exercise Journal

Weight Training

REPETITION SCHEME _____   REST INTERVALS _____

DATE _____   TIME _____   PRE-WORKOUT ENERGY LEVEL _____

Muscle Group	Exercise	Warm-up	Set 1	Set 2	Set 3	Set 4

Cardiovascular Exercise

Type	Total Cardio Time	Time in HR Range	Heart Rate
Bike			
Treadmill			
Stairclimber			
Run			
Aerobics class			
Other			

Nutrition Journal

DATE _____   WEEK _____   DAY _____

Meal Time	Meal	Foods	Total Calories	Grams Protein	Grams Carbs	Grams Fat	Meal Comments
_____ am/pm	1						
			_____ total	_____ total	_____ total	_____ total	
_____ am/pm	2						
			_____ total	_____ total	_____ total	_____ total	
_____ am/pm	3						
			_____ total	_____ total	_____ total	_____ total	
_____ am/pm	4						
			_____ total	_____ total	_____ total	_____ total	
_____ am/pm	5						
			_____ total	_____ total	_____ total	_____ total	

Exercise Journal

Weight Training

REPETITION SCHEME _____   REST INTERVALS _____
DATE _____   TIME _____   PRE-WORKOUT ENERGY LEVEL _____

Muscle Group	Exercise	Warm-up	Set 1	Set 2	Set 3	Set 4

Cardiovascular Exercise

Type	Total Cardio Time	Time in HR Range	Heart Rate
Bike			
Treadmill			
Stairclimber			
Run			
Aerobics class			
Other			

Nutrition Journal

DATE _____   WEEK _____   DAY _____

Meal Time	Meal	Foods	Total Calories	Grams Protein	Grams Carbs	Grams Fat	Meal Comments
_____ am/pm	1						
			_____ total	_____ total	_____ total	_____ total	
_____ am/pm	2						
			_____ total	_____ total	_____ total	_____ total	
_____ am/pm	3						
			_____ total	_____ total	_____ total	_____ total	
_____ am/pm	4						
			_____ total	_____ total	_____ total	_____ total	
_____ am/pm	5						
			_____ total	_____ total	_____ total	_____ total	

Exercise Journal

Weight Training

REPETITION SCHEME _____   REST INTERVALS _____
DATE _____   TIME _____   PRE-WORKOUT ENERGY LEVEL _____

Muscle Group	Exercise	Warm-up	Set 1	Set 2	Set 3	Set 4

Cardiovascular Exercise

Type	Total Cardio Time	Time in HR Range	Heart Rate
Bike			
Treadmill			
Stairclimber			
Run			
Aerobics class			
Other			

Nutrition Journal

DATE _____   WEEK _____   DAY _____

Meal Time	Meal	Foods	Total Calories	Grams Protein	Grams Carbs	Grams Fat	Meal Comments
_____ am/pm	1						
			_____ total	_____ total	_____ total	_____ total	
_____ am/pm	2						
			_____ total	_____ total	_____ total	_____ total	
_____ am/pm	3						
			_____ total	_____ total	_____ total	_____ total	
_____ am/pm	4						
			_____ total	_____ total	_____ total	_____ total	
_____ am/pm	5						
			_____ total	_____ total	_____ total	_____ total	

Exercise Journal

Weight Training

REPETITION SCHEME _____   REST INTERVALS _____
DATE _____   TIME _____   PRE-WORKOUT ENERGY LEVEL _____

Muscle Group	Exercise	Warm-up	Set 1	Set 2	Set 3	Set 4

Cardiovascular Exercise

Type	Total Cardio Time	Time in HR Range	Heart Rate
Bike			
Treadmill			
Stairclimber			
Run			
Aerobics class			
Other			

Nutrition Journal

DATE _____   WEEK _____   DAY _____

Meal Time	Meal	Foods	Total Calories	Grams Protein	Grams Carbs	Grams Fat	Meal Comments
_____ am/pm	1		_____ total	_____ total	_____ total	_____ total	
_____ am/pm	2		_____ total	_____ total	_____ total	_____ total	
_____ am/pm	3		_____ total	_____ total	_____ total	_____ total	
_____ am/pm	4		_____ total	_____ total	_____ total	_____ total	
_____ am/pm	5		_____ total	_____ total	_____ total	_____ total	

Exercise Journal

Weight Training

REPETITION SCHEME _____   REST INTERVALS _____
DATE _____   TIME _____   PRE-WORKOUT ENERGY LEVEL _____

Muscle Group	Exercise	Warm-up	Set 1	Set 2	Set 3	Set 4

Cardiovascular Exercise

Type	Total Cardio Time	Time in HR Range	Heart Rate
Bike			
Treadmill			
Stairclimber			
Run			
Aerobics class			
Other			

Nutrition Journal

DATE _____   WEEK _____   DAY _____

Meal Time	Meal	Foods	Total Calories	Grams Protein	Grams Carbs	Grams Fat	Meal Comments
_____ am/pm	1						
			_____ total	_____ total	_____ total	_____ total	
_____ am/pm	2						
			_____ total	_____ total	_____ total	_____ total	
_____ am/pm	3						
			_____ total	_____ total	_____ total	_____ total	
_____ am/pm	4						
			_____ total	_____ total	_____ total	_____ total	
_____ am/pm	5						
			_____ total	_____ total	_____ total	_____ total	

Exercise Journal

Weight Training

REPETITION SCHEME _____   REST INTERVALS _____
DATE _____   TIME _____   PRE-WORKOUT ENERGY LEVEL _____

Muscle Group	Exercise	Warm-up	Set 1	Set 2	Set 3	Set 4

Cardiovascular Exercise

Type	Total Cardio Time	Time in HR Range	Heart Rate
Bike			
Treadmill			
Stairclimber			
Run			
Aerobics class			
Other			

Nutrition Journal

DATE _____   WEEK _____   DAY _____

Meal Time	Meal	Foods	Total Calories	Grams Protein	Grams Carbs	Grams Fat	Meal Comments
_____ am/pm	1						
			_____ total	_____ total	_____ total	_____ total	
_____ am/pm	2						
			_____ total	_____ total	_____ total	_____ total	
_____ am/pm	3						
			_____ total	_____ total	_____ total	_____ total	
_____ am/pm	4						
			_____ total	_____ total	_____ total	_____ total	
_____ am/pm	5						
			_____ total	_____ total	_____ total	_____ total	

Exercise Journal

Weight Training

REPETITION SCHEME _____   REST INTERVALS _____
DATE _____   TIME _____   PRE-WORKOUT ENERGY LEVEL _____

Muscle Group	Exercise	Warm-up	Set 1	Set 2	Set 3	Set 4

Cardiovascular Exercise

Type	Total Cardio Time	Time in HR Range	Heart Rate
Bike			
Treadmill			
Stairclimber			
Run			
Aerobics class			
Other			

Nutrition Journal

DATE _____   WEEK _____   DAY _____

Meal Time	Meal	Foods	Total Calories	Grams Protein	Grams Carbs	Grams Fat	Meal Comments
_____ am/pm	1						
			_____ total	_____ total	_____ total	_____ total	
_____ am/pm	2						
			_____ total	_____ total	_____ total	_____ total	
_____ am/pm	3						
			_____ total	_____ total	_____ total	_____ total	
_____ am/pm	4						
			_____ total	_____ total	_____ total	_____ total	
_____ am/pm	5						
			_____ total	_____ total	_____ total	_____ total	

Exercise Journal

Weight Training

REPETITION SCHEME _____   REST INTERVALS _____
DATE _____   TIME _____   PRE-WORKOUT ENERGY LEVEL _____

Muscle Group	Exercise	Warm-up	Set 1	Set 2	Set 3	Set 4

Cardiovascular Exercise

Type	Total Cardio Time	Time in HR Range	Heart Rate
Bike			
Treadmill			
Stairclimber			
Run			
Aerobics class			
Other			

Nutrition Journal

DATE _____   WEEK _____   DAY _____

Meal Time	Meal	Foods	Total Calories	Grams Protein	Grams Carbs	Grams Fat	Meal Comments
_____ am/pm	1						
			_____ total	_____ total	_____ total	_____ total	
_____ am/pm	2						
			_____ total	_____ total	_____ total	_____ total	
_____ am/pm	3						
			_____ total	_____ total	_____ total	_____ total	
_____ am/pm	4						
			_____ total	_____ total	_____ total	_____ total	
_____ am/pm	5						
			_____ total	_____ total	_____ total	_____ total	

Exercise Journal

Weight Training

REPETITION SCHEME _____   REST INTERVALS _____
DATE _____   TIME _____   PRE-WORKOUT ENERGY LEVEL _____

Muscle Group	Exercise	Warm-up	Set 1	Set 2	Set 3	Set 4

Cardiovascular Exercise

Type	Total Cardio Time	Time in HR Range	Heart Rate
Bike			
Treadmill			
Stairclimber			
Run			
Aerobics class			
Other			

Nutrition Journal

DATE _____   WEEK _____   DAY _____

Meal Time	Meal	Foods	Total Calories	Grams Protein	Grams Carbs	Grams Fat	Meal Comments
_____ am/pm	1						
			_____ total	_____ total	_____ total	_____ total	
_____ am/pm	2						
			_____ total	_____ total	_____ total	_____ total	
_____ am/pm	3						
			_____ total	_____ total	_____ total	_____ total	
_____ am/pm	4						
			_____ total	_____ total	_____ total	_____ total	
_____ am/pm	5						
			_____ total	_____ total	_____ total	_____ total	

Exercise Journal

Weight Training

REPETITION SCHEME _____   REST INTERVALS _____
DATE _____   TIME _____   PRE-WORKOUT ENERGY LEVEL _____

Muscle Group	Exercise	Warm-up	Set 1	Set 2	Set 3	Set 4

Cardiovascular Exercise

Type	Total Cardio Time	Time in HR Range	Heart Rate
Bike			
Treadmill			
Stairclimber			
Run			
Aerobics class			
Other			

Nutrition Journal

DATE _____   WEEK _____   DAY _____

Meal Time	Meal	Foods	Total Calories	Grams Protein	Grams Carbs	Grams Fat	Meal Comments
_____ am/pm	1						
			_____ total	_____ total	_____ total	_____ total	
_____ am/pm	2						
			_____ total	_____ total	_____ total	_____ total	
_____ am/pm	3						
			_____ total	_____ total	_____ total	_____ total	
_____ am/pm	4						
			_____ total	_____ total	_____ total	_____ total	
_____ am/pm	5						
			_____ total	_____ total	_____ total	_____ total	

Exercise Journal

Weight Training

REPETITION SCHEME _____   REST INTERVALS _____
DATE _____   TIME _____   PRE-WORKOUT ENERGY LEVEL _____

Muscle Group	Exercise	Warm-up	Set 1	Set 2	Set 3	Set 4

Cardiovascular Exercise

Type	Total Cardio Time	Time in HR Range	Heart Rate
Bike			
Treadmill			
Stairclimber			
Run			
Aerobics class			
Other			

Nutrition Journal

DATE _____   WEEK _____   DAY _____

Meal Time	Meal	Foods	Total Calories	Grams Protein	Grams Carbs	Grams Fat	Meal Comments
_____ am/pm	1						
			total	total	total	total	
_____ am/pm	2						
			total	total	total	total	
_____ am/pm	3						
			total	total	total	total	
_____ am/pm	4						
			total	total	total	total	
_____ am/pm	5						
			total	total	total	total	

Exercise Journal

Weight Training

REPETITION SCHEME _____   REST INTERVALS _____
DATE _____   TIME _____   PRE-WORKOUT ENERGY LEVEL _____

Muscle Group	Exercise	Warm-up	Set 1	Set 2	Set 3	Set 4

Cardiovascular Exercise

Type	Total Cardio Time	Time in HR Range	Heart Rate
Bike			
Treadmill			
Stairclimber			
Run			
Aerobics class			
Other			

Nutrition Journal

DATE _____   WEEK _____   DAY _____

Meal Time	Meal	Foods	Total Calories	Grams Protein	Grams Carbs	Grams Fat	Meal Comments
_____ am/pm	1						
			_____ total	_____ total	_____ total	_____ total	
_____ am/pm	2						
			_____ total	_____ total	_____ total	_____ total	
_____ am/pm	3						
			_____ total	_____ total	_____ total	_____ total	
_____ am/pm	4						
			_____ total	_____ total	_____ total	_____ total	
_____ am/pm	5						
			_____ total	_____ total	_____ total	_____ total	

Exercise Journal

Weight Training

REPETITION SCHEME _____   REST INTERVALS _____

DATE _____   TIME _____   PRE-WORKOUT ENERGY LEVEL _____

Muscle Group	Exercise	Warm-up	Set 1	Set 2	Set 3	Set 4

Cardiovascular Exercise

Type	Total Cardio Time	Time in HR Range	Heart Rate
Bike			
Treadmill			
Stairclimber			
Run			
Aerobics class			
Other			

Nutrition Journal

DATE _____   WEEK _____   DAY _____

Meal Time	Meal	Foods	Total Calories	Grams Protein	Grams Carbs	Grams Fat	Meal Comments
_____ am/pm	1		____ total	____ total	____ total	____ total	
_____ am/pm	2		____ total	____ total	____ total	____ total	
_____ am/pm	3		____ total	____ total	____ total	____ total	
_____ am/pm	4		____ total	____ total	____ total	____ total	
_____ am/pm	5		____ total	____ total	____ total	____ total	

Exercise Journal

Weight Training

REPETITION SCHEME _____   REST INTERVALS _____
DATE _____   TIME _____   PRE-WORKOUT ENERGY LEVEL _____

Muscle Group	Exercise	Warm-up	Set 1	Set 2	Set 3	Set 4

Cardiovascular Exercise

Type	Total Cardio Time	Time in HR Range	Heart Rate
Bike			
Treadmill			
Stairclimber			
Run			
Aerobics class			
Other			

Nutrition Journal

DATE _____   WEEK _____   DAY _____

Meal Time	Meal	Foods	Total Calories	Grams Protein	Grams Carbs	Grams Fat	Meal Comments
_____ am/pm	1						
			total	total	total	total	
_____ am/pm	2						
			total	total	total	total	
_____ am/pm	3						
			total	total	total	total	
_____ am/pm	4						
			total	total	total	total	
_____ am/pm	5						
			total	total	total	total	

Exercise Journal

Weight Training

REPETITION SCHEME _____   REST INTERVALS _____
DATE _____   TIME _____   PRE-WORKOUT ENERGY LEVEL _____

Muscle Group	Exercise	Warm-up	Set 1	Set 2	Set 3	Set 4

Cardiovascular Exercise

Type	Total Cardio Time	Time in HR Range	Heart Rate
Bike			
Treadmill			
Stairclimber			
Run			
Aerobics class			
Other			

Nutrition Journal

DATE _____   WEEK _____   DAY _____

Meal Time	Meal	Foods	Total Calories	Grams Protein	Grams Carbs	Grams Fat	Meal Comments
_____ am/pm	1		___ total	___ total	___ total	___ total	
_____ am/pm	2		___ total	___ total	___ total	___ total	
_____ am/pm	3		___ total	___ total	___ total	___ total	
_____ am/pm	4		___ total	___ total	___ total	___ total	
_____ am/pm	5		___ total	___ total	___ total	___ total	

Exercise Journal

Weight Training

REPETITION SCHEME _____   REST INTERVALS _____
DATE _____   TIME _____   PRE-WORKOUT ENERGY LEVEL _____

Muscle Group	Exercise	Warm-up	Set 1	Set 2	Set 3	Set 4

Cardiovascular Exercise

Type	Total Cardio Time	Time in HR Range	Heart Rate
Bike			
Treadmill			
Stairclimber			
Run			
Aerobics class			
Other			

Nutrition Journal

DATE _____   WEEK _____   DAY _____

Meal Time	Meal	Foods	Total Calories	Grams Protein	Grams Carbs	Grams Fat	Meal Comments
_____ am/pm	1		_____ total	_____ total	_____ total	_____ total	
_____ am/pm	2		_____ total	_____ total	_____ total	_____ total	
_____ am/pm	3		_____ total	_____ total	_____ total	_____ total	
_____ am/pm	4		_____ total	_____ total	_____ total	_____ total	
_____ am/pm	5		_____ total	_____ total	_____ total	_____ total	

Exercise Journal

Weight Training

REPETITION SCHEME _____   REST INTERVALS _____
DATE _____   TIME _____   PRE-WORKOUT ENERGY LEVEL _____

Muscle Group	Exercise	Warm-up	Set 1	Set 2	Set 3	Set 4

Cardiovascular Exercise

Type	Total Cardio Time	Time in HR Range	Heart Rate
Bike			
Treadmill			
Stairclimber			
Run			
Aerobics class			
Other			

Nutrition Journal

DATE _____   WEEK _____   DAY _____

Meal Time	Meal	Foods	Total Calories	Grams Protein	Grams Carbs	Grams Fat	Meal Comments
_____ am/pm	1						
			_____ total	_____ total	_____ total	_____ total	
_____ am/pm	2						
			_____ total	_____ total	_____ total	_____ total	
_____ am/pm	3						
			_____ total	_____ total	_____ total	_____ total	
_____ am/pm	4						
			_____ total	_____ total	_____ total	_____ total	
_____ am/pm	5						
			_____ total	_____ total	_____ total	_____ total	

Exercise Journal

Weight Training

REPETITION SCHEME _____   REST INTERVALS _____
DATE _____   TIME _____   PRE-WORKOUT ENERGY LEVEL _____

Muscle Group	Exercise	Warm-up	Set 1	Set 2	Set 3	Set 4

Cardiovascular Exercise

Type	Total Cardio Time	Time in HR Range	Heart Rate
Bike			
Treadmill			
Stairclimber			
Run			
Aerobics class			
Other			

Nutrition Journal

DATE _____   WEEK _____   DAY _____

Meal Time	Meal	Foods	Total Calories	Grams Protein	Grams Carbs	Grams Fat	Meal Comments
_____ am/pm	1						
			_____ total	_____ total	_____ total	_____ total	
_____ am/pm	2						
			_____ total	_____ total	_____ total	_____ total	
_____ am/pm	3						
			_____ total	_____ total	_____ total	_____ total	
_____ am/pm	4						
			_____ total	_____ total	_____ total	_____ total	
_____ am/pm	5						
			_____ total	_____ total	_____ total	_____ total	

Exercise Journal

Weight Training

REPETITION SCHEME _____   REST INTERVALS _____
DATE _____   TIME _____   PRE-WORKOUT ENERGY LEVEL _____

Muscle Group	Exercise	Warm-up	Set 1	Set 2	Set 3	Set 4

Cardiovascular Exercise

Type	Total Cardio Time	Time in HR Range	Heart Rate
Bike			
Treadmill			
Stairclimber			
Run			
Aerobics class			
Other			

Nutrition Journal

DATE _____   WEEK _____   DAY _____

Meal Time	Meal	Foods	Total Calories	Grams Protein	Grams Carbs	Grams Fat	Meal Comments
_____ am/pm	1						
			_____ total	_____ total	_____ total	_____ total	
_____ am/pm	2						
			_____ total	_____ total	_____ total	_____ total	
_____ am/pm	3						
			_____ total	_____ total	_____ total	_____ total	
_____ am/pm	4						
			_____ total	_____ total	_____ total	_____ total	
_____ am/pm	5						
			_____ total	_____ total	_____ total	_____ total	

Exercise Journal

Weight Training

REPETITION SCHEME _____   REST INTERVALS _____
DATE _____   TIME _____   PRE-WORKOUT ENERGY LEVEL _____

Muscle Group	Exercise	Warm-up	Set 1	Set 2	Set 3	Set 4

Cardiovascular Exercise

Type	Total Cardio Time	Time in HR Range	Heart Rate
Bike			
Treadmill			
Stairclimber			
Run			
Aerobics class			
Other			

Nutrition Journal

DATE _____   WEEK _____   DAY _____

Meal Time	Meal	Foods	Total Calories	Grams Protein	Grams Carbs	Grams Fat	Meal Comments
_____ am/pm	1						
			_____ total	_____ total	_____ total	_____ total	
_____ am/pm	2						
			_____ total	_____ total	_____ total	_____ total	
_____ am/pm	3						
			_____ total	_____ total	_____ total	_____ total	
_____ am/pm	4						
			_____ total	_____ total	_____ total	_____ total	
_____ am/pm	5						
			_____ total	_____ total	_____ total	_____ total	

Exercise Journal

Weight Training

REPETITION SCHEME _____   REST INTERVALS _____
DATE _____   TIME _____   PRE-WORKOUT ENERGY LEVEL _____

Muscle Group	Exercise	Warm-up	Set 1	Set 2	Set 3	Set 4

Cardiovascular Exercise

Type	Total Cardio Time	Time in HR Range	Heart Rate
Bike			
Treadmill			
Stairclimber			
Run			
Aerobics class			
Other			

Nutrition Journal

DATE _____   WEEK _____   DAY _____

Meal Time	Meal	Foods	Total Calories	Grams Protein	Grams Carbs	Grams Fat	Meal Comments
_____ am/pm	1						
			_____ total	_____ total	_____ total	_____ total	
_____ am/pm	2						
			_____ total	_____ total	_____ total	_____ total	
_____ am/pm	3						
			_____ total	_____ total	_____ total	_____ total	
_____ am/pm	4						
			_____ total	_____ total	_____ total	_____ total	
_____ am/pm	5						
			_____ total	_____ total	_____ total	_____ total	

Exercise Journal

Weight Training

REPETITION SCHEME _____   REST INTERVALS _____
DATE _____   TIME _____   PRE-WORKOUT ENERGY LEVEL _____

Muscle Group	Exercise	Warm-up	Set 1	Set 2	Set 3	Set 4

Cardiovascular Exercise

Type	Total Cardio Time	Time in HR Range	Heart Rate
Bike			
Treadmill			
Stairclimber			
Run			
Aerobics class			
Other			

Nutrition Journal

DATE _____   WEEK _____   DAY _____

Meal Time	Meal	Foods	Total Calories	Grams Protein	Grams Carbs	Grams Fat	Meal Comments
_____ am/pm	1						
			_____ total	_____ total	_____ total	_____ total	
_____ am/pm	2						
			_____ total	_____ total	_____ total	_____ total	
_____ am/pm	3						
			_____ total	_____ total	_____ total	_____ total	
_____ am/pm	4						
			_____ total	_____ total	_____ total	_____ total	
_____ am/pm	5						
			_____ total	_____ total	_____ total	_____ total	

Exercise Journal

Weight Training

REPETITION SCHEME _____   REST INTERVALS _____
DATE _____   TIME _____   PRE-WORKOUT ENERGY LEVEL _____

Muscle Group	Exercise	Warm-up	Set 1	Set 2	Set 3	Set 4

Cardiovascular Exercise

Type	Total Cardio Time	Time in HR Range	Heart Rate
Bike			
Treadmill			
Stairclimber			
Run			
Aerobics class			
Other			

Nutrition Journal

DATE _____   WEEK _____   DAY _____

Meal Time	Meal	Foods	Total Calories	Grams Protein	Grams Carbs	Grams Fat	Meal Comments
_____ am/pm	1						
			_____ total	_____ total	_____ total	_____ total	
_____ am/pm	2						
			_____ total	_____ total	_____ total	_____ total	
_____ am/pm	3						
			_____ total	_____ total	_____ total	_____ total	
_____ am/pm	4						
			_____ total	_____ total	_____ total	_____ total	
_____ am/pm	5						
			_____ total	_____ total	_____ total	_____ total	

Exercise Journal

Weight Training

REPETITION SCHEME _____   REST INTERVALS _____
DATE _____   TIME _____   PRE-WORKOUT ENERGY LEVEL _____

Muscle Group	Exercise	Warm-up	Set 1	Set 2	Set 3	Set 4

Cardiovascular Exercise

Type	Total Cardio Time	Time in HR Range	Heart Rate
Bike			
Treadmill			
Stairclimber			
Run			
Aerobics class			
Other			

Nutrition Journal

DATE _____   WEEK _____   DAY _____

Meal Time	Meal	Foods	Total Calories	Grams Protein	Grams Carbs	Grams Fat	Meal Comments
_____ am/pm	1						
			_____ total	_____ total	_____ total	_____ total	
_____ am/pm	2						
			_____ total	_____ total	_____ total	_____ total	
_____ am/pm	3						
			_____ total	_____ total	_____ total	_____ total	
_____ am/pm	4						
			_____ total	_____ total	_____ total	_____ total	
_____ am/pm	5						
			_____ total	_____ total	_____ total	_____ total	

Exercise Journal

Weight Training

REPETITION SCHEME _____   REST INTERVALS _____
DATE _____   TIME _____   PRE-WORKOUT ENERGY LEVEL _____

Muscle Group	Exercise	Warm-up	Set 1	Set 2	Set 3	Set 4

Cardiovascular Exercise

Type	Total Cardio Time	Time in HR Range	Heart Rate
Bike			
Treadmill			
Stairclimber			
Run			
Aerobics class			
Other			

Nutrition Journal

DATE _____   WEEK _____   DAY _____

Meal Time	Meal	Foods	Total Calories	Grams Protein	Grams Carbs	Grams Fat	Meal Comments
_____ am/pm	1						
			_____ total	_____ total	_____ total	_____ total	
_____ am/pm	2						
			_____ total	_____ total	_____ total	_____ total	
_____ am/pm	3						
			_____ total	_____ total	_____ total	_____ total	
_____ am/pm	4						
			_____ total	_____ total	_____ total	_____ total	
_____ am/pm	5						
			_____ total	_____ total	_____ total	_____ total	

Exercise Journal

Weight Training

REPETITION SCHEME _____   REST INTERVALS _____
DATE _____   TIME _____   PRE-WORKOUT ENERGY LEVEL _____

Muscle Group	Exercise	Warm-up	Set 1	Set 2	Set 3	Set 4

Cardiovascular Exercise

Type	Total Cardio Time	Time in HR Range	Heart Rate
Bike			
Treadmill			
Stairclimber			
Run			
Aerobics class			
Other			

Nutrition Journal

DATE _____   WEEK _____   DAY _____

Meal Time	Meal	Foods	Total Calories	Grams Protein	Grams Carbs	Grams Fat	Meal Comments
_____ am/pm	1		____ total	____ total	____ total	____ total	
_____ am/pm	2		____ total	____ total	____ total	____ total	
_____ am/pm	3		____ total	____ total	____ total	____ total	
_____ am/pm	4		____ total	____ total	____ total	____ total	
_____ am/pm	5		____ total	____ total	____ total	____ total	

Exercise Journal

Weight Training

REPETITION SCHEME _____   REST INTERVALS _____
DATE _____   TIME _____   PRE-WORKOUT ENERGY LEVEL _____

Muscle Group	Exercise	Warm-up	Set 1	Set 2	Set 3	Set 4

Cardiovascular Exercise

Type	Total Cardio Time	Time in HR Range	Heart Rate
Bike			
Treadmill			
Stairclimber			
Run			
Aerobics class			
Other			

APPENDIX:

FOOD NUTRITION VALUES

The following tables provide you with the nutritional breakdown of protein, carbohydrates, and fat in various foods. The protein and carbohydrate groups are subdivided.

Use these tables to help you create your meals.

Group IA: Protein—with Fat

Group IB: Protein—Lean

Group IC: Protein—Lean Dairy

Group ID: Protein—Dairy with Fat

Group IIA: Carbohydrates—Vegetables

Group IIB: Carbohydrates—Fruits

Group IIC: Carbohydrates—Grains, etc.

Group III: Fat

Group IV: Fast Foods

Group IA
Protein—with Fat

Beef

Type	Serving	Calories	P (gm)	C (gm)	F (gm)
Bottom round	2.0 oz	110	12	—	7
Flank steak	2.0 oz	102	11	—	6
Ground beef (extra lean)	1.5 oz	99	8	—	7
Ground beef (lean)	1.25 oz	94	6	—	7
Ground beef (regular)	1.25 oz	110	6	—	9
Rib eye	1.25 oz	98	6	—	8
Round tip	1.75 oz	100	10	—	6
T-bone	1.25 oz	100	6	—	8
Top round	2.0 oz	100	12	—	5
Top sirloin	1.5 oz	93	8	—	6

Cheese

American	1.0 oz	110	6	1	9
Blue	1.0 oz	100	6	1	9
Brie	1.25 oz	101	6	—	8
Cheddar	1.0 oz	110	7	1	9
Colby	1.0 oz	110	7	1	9
Cream cheese	1.0 oz	100	2	1	10
Monterey jack	1.0 oz	110	6	—	9
Mozzarella (part skim)	1.25 oz	100	10	1	6
Mozzarella (whole)	1.0 oz	90	6	1	7
Muenster	1.0 oz	100	7	—	9
Parmesan (grated)	.75 oz	98	9	1	7
Provolone	1.0 oz	100	7	1	7
Ricotta (low fat)	2.25 oz	101	7	2	7
Ricotta (whole)	2.0 oz	100	7	2	7
Romano (grated)	.75 oz	98	8	1	7
String (mozzarella, part skim)	1.25 oz	100	10	1	6
Swiss	1.0 oz	110	8	1	8

Eggs

Egg, whole (large)	1.25 eggs	100	8	—	7
Egg yolk	1.5 yolks	90	4	—	8

Group IA cont.

Seafood

Type	Serving	Calories	P (gm)	C (gm)	F (gm)
Eel	2.0 oz	104	10	—	7
Herring	2.25 oz	101	11	—	6
Orange roughy	3.0 oz	108	13	—	6
Salmon	2.5 oz	100	14	—	5
Sardines (mustard sauce)	1.75 oz	103	7	1	7
Tuna (solid in oil)	2.0 oz	100	14	—	8

Turkey

Ground turkey (93% fat free)	2.25 oz	104	16	—	5

Group IB

Protein—Lean

Cheese

Type	Serving	Calories	P (gm)	C (gm)	F (gm)
Cheddar (fat free)	2.5 oz	100	23	3	—
Cottage cheese (fat free)	6.0 oz	105	23	5	—
Cottage cheese (low fat)	4.0 oz	100	14	4	2
Cottage cheese (regular)	3.5 oz	89	12	3	4
Cream cheese (fat free)	4.0 oz	100	16	4	—
Mozzarella (fat free)	2.5 oz	100	23	3	—

Chicken

Chicken breast (boneless/skinless)	3.5 oz	109	23	—	1
Chicken breast (canned in water)	2.5 oz	100	15	—	4
Chicken breast (lunch meat 99% fat free)	3.5 oz	105	18	—	—
Chicken drumstick	3 oz	102	17	—	3

continued

Group IB cont.

Eggs

Type	Serving	Calories	P (gm)	C (gm)	F (gm)
Egg white (packaged)	1 cup	100	20	4	—
Egg white (large)	6	102	23	—	1

Seafood

Type	Serving	Calories	P (gm)	C (gm)	F (gm)
Bass, sea	4.0 oz	108	21	—	3
Bass, striped	4.0 oz	108	21	—	3
Catfish	4.0 oz	108	19	—	3
Clams (steamed)	2.5 oz	105	18	—	1
Cod	4.5 oz	104	23	1	—
Crab	4.0 oz	102	22	—	2
Crab cake	2.5 oz	105	19	—	2
Flounder	4.5 oz	101	21	—	1
Halibut	3.25 oz	101	19	—	2
Lobster	4.0 oz	111	23	2	1
Mahimahi	4.0 oz	96	21	—	1
Mussels	2.0 oz	98	13	4	3
Octopus	4.5 oz	104	19	3	1
Oysters	4.5 oz	104	12	6	3
Pollack	4.0 oz	104	22	—	1
Salmon (lean)	3.5 oz	105	18	—	4
Shark	2.75 oz	102	16	—	4
Shrimp	4.0 oz	112	24	—	1
Snapper	3.5 oz	98	20	—	1
Sole	4.0 oz	104	21	—	1
Swordfish	3.0 oz	102	17	—	3
Trout	3.5 oz	102	16	—	4
Tuna (fresh)	3.5 oz	109	23	—	1
Tuna (solid in water)	3.5 oz	105	25	—	4
Whitefish	2.5 oz	95	14	—	4
Yellowtail	2.5 oz	103	17	—	4

Turkey

Type	Serving	Calories	P (gm)	C (gm)	F (gm)
Ground turkey breast (99% fat free)	3.5 oz	105	25	—	1

Protein—Lean Dairy

Milk

Type	Serving	Calories	P (gm)	C (gm)	F (gm)
Milk, 1%	8.0 oz	104	8	12	3
Milk, nonfat	8.0 oz	88	9	12	1
Milk, 1% (lactose reduced)	10.0 oz	100	10	7	3
Milk, nonfat (lactose reduced)	10.0 oz	100	10	16	—

Yogurt

Type	Serving	Calories	P (gm)	C (gm)	F (gm)
Frozen yogurt (nonfat)	3.5 oz	99	4	21	—
Frozen yogurt (sugar free, nonfat)	10.0 oz	100	5	23	—
Yogurt, plain (nonfat)	7.0 oz	98	10	14	—
Yogurt, vanilla (low fat)	3.5 oz	105	5	19	2
Yogurt, vanilla (nonfat)	8.0 oz	100	9	16	—

Cheese

Type	Serving	Calories	P (gm)	C (gm)	F (gm)
Parmesan (grated fat free)	1.25 oz	108	14	14	—
Ricotta (fat free)	4.0 oz	90	18	6	—
Swiss (fat free)	2.5 oz	100	15	10	—

Protein—Dairy with Fat

Milk

Type	Serving	Calories	P (gm)	C (gm)	F (gm)
Milk, 2% low fat	8.0 oz	120	8	12	5
Milk, 2% low fat (lactose reduced)	6.0 oz	96	6	9	4
Milk, whole	6.0 oz	113	6	8	6

Yogurt

Type	Serving	Calories	P (gm)	C (gm)	F (gm)
Frozen yogurt (low fat)	3.0 oz	101	3	18	3
Yogurt, plain (low fat)	5.0 oz	100	8	11	3
Yogurt, plain (whole)	4.0 oz	100	6	8	5
Yogurt, vanilla (whole)	4.0 oz	108	4	15	4

Group IIA
Carbohydrates—Vegetables

Type	Serving	Calories	P (gm)	C (gm)	F (gm)
Alfalfa sprouts	6.0 oz	48	7	7	1
Artichoke hearts (boiled)	4.0 oz	57	4	13	—
Asparagus	8.0 oz	48	7	8	1
Bamboo shoots	6.0 oz	48	4	9	1
Bean sprouts	16.0 oz	48	6	11	1
Black-eyed peas	2.0 oz	52	2	11	—
Beets, pickled (canned)	¼ cup	40	1	10	—
Broccoli	6.0 oz	48	5	9	1
Brussels sprouts	4.0 oz	48	4	10	—
Cabbage	7.0 oz	49	2	11	1
Carrot	4.0 oz	48	1	11	2
Carrot juice	¼ cup	52	1	9	—
Cauliflower	7.0 oz	49	4	10	—
Celery	10.0 oz	50	2	10	—
Chives	7.0 oz	49	6	8	1
Coleslaw	½ cup	41	1	7	2
Collards	5.0 oz	45	2	10	1
Cucumber	13.0 oz	52	3	10	1
Eggplant	7.0 oz	49	2	13	1
Garbanzo beans	.50 oz	51	3	9	1
Garden salad	medium	50	4	10	—
Green beans (canned)	1.0 cup	40	2	8	1
Hummus	1.0 oz	48	1	6	2
Kale	3.5 oz	49	3	10	1
Kidney beans (canned)	¼ cup	45	4	10	1
Leek	3.0 oz	51	1	12	—
Lentil	.50 oz	48	4	8	—
Lettuce	10.0 oz	40	4	7	1
Lima beans (canned)	¼ cup	40	3	8	—
Lima beans (frozen)	¼ cup	50	3	9	—
Lima beans (raw)	1.5 oz	48	3	9	—
Mushroom, shiitake	.50 oz	42	1	11	—
Mushroom, white	7.0 oz	49	4	9	1
Navy beans (canned)	6.0 oz	53	5	14	—
Navy beans (raw)	.50 oz	48	3	9	—
Okra	4.0 oz	44	2	9	—
Onion	4.0 oz	44	1	10	—
Parsley (dried)	.50 oz	40	3	7	1
Parsnips	2.5 oz	53	1	13	—

Group IIA cont.

Type	Serving	Calories	P (gm)	C (gm)	F (gm)
Peas, green (canned)	½ cup	50	3	12	—
Peas, green (frozen)	½ cup	60	4	12	1
Peas, green (raw)	2.0 oz	46	3	8	—
Peppers, green/red	7.0 oz	48	2	11	1
Peppers, jalepeño	5.0 oz	50	—	15	—
Peppers, sweet	6.0 oz	48	2	11	—
Pickles, dill	10.0 oz	40	—	10	—
Pickles, sweet	1.5 oz	53	—	12	—
Pinto beans (canned)	¼ cup	45	3	10	1
Pinto beans (raw)	.50 oz	48	3	9	—
Pumpkin (canned)	½ cup	35	1	9	—
Radish	10.0 oz	50	2	10	2
Red beans (canned)	¼ cup	45	3	9	1
Relish, hamburger	1.0 oz	40	—	9	—
Rutabaga	5.0 oz	50	2	12	1
Sauerkraut (canned)	1.0 cup	50	2	12	—
Snowpeas	4.0 oz	48	3	8	—
Spinach (canned)	1.0 cup	50	6	7	1
Spinach (frozen)	1.0 cup	50	8	10	—
Spinach (raw)	9.0 oz	54	7	9	1
Squash, acorn	4.0 oz	44	1	12	—
Squash, banana	3.0 oz	54	2	13	—
Squash, butternut	4.0 oz	52	1	13	—
Squash, summer	9.0 oz	54	3	11	1
Squash, winter	4.0 oz	44	2	10	—
Succotash (frozen)	¼ cup	37	2	8	—
Tofu	2.0 oz	44	5	1	3
Tomato (canned/whole)	1.0 cup	50	2	12	1
Tomato (raw)	9.0 oz	54	2	12	1
Tomato juice	6.0 oz	40	1	8	—
Tomato paste	2.0 oz	50	2	11	—
Tomato sauce	1.0 cup	60	4	12	—
Turnips (canned)	1.0 cup	42	4	6	1
Turnips (raw)	6.0 oz	48	2	11	1
Vegetable juice (canned)	1.0 cup	47	1	11	—
Vegetables, mixed (frozen)	½ cup	40	2	9	—
Water chestnut	1.5 oz	45	1	10	1
Wax beans (canned)	1.0 cup	40	—	8	—

continued

Group IIA cont.

Type	Serving	Calories	P (gm)	C (gm)	F (gm)
White beans (canned)	2.0 oz	38	2	7	—
White beans (raw)	.50 oz	47	3	9	—
Zucchini (frozen)	10.0 oz	48	3	10	—
Zucchini (raw)	12.0 oz	48	4	10	—

Group IIB
Carbohydrates—Fruits

Type	Serving	Calories	P (gm)	C (gm)	F (gm)
Apple	9.0 oz	153	1	39	1
Apple (dried)	2.0 oz	150	1	42	—
Apple butter (unsweetened)	4.5 tbsp	149	—	42	—
Apple cider	10.0 oz	150	—	35	—
Apple juice	12.0 oz	160	—	40	—
Applesauce (unsweetened)	1.5 cups	150	—	36	—
Apricot	1.0 oz	154	4	35	1
Apricot (dried)	2.0 oz	140	2	35	—
Apricot nectar	9.0 oz	150	2	39	—
Banana	6.0 oz	156	1	41	—
Blackberry	2.0 cups	148	2	37	—
Blueberry	9.0 oz	144	2	36	1
Boysenberry (frozen)	2.25 cups	149	3	36	1
Cantaloupe (meat only)	15.0 oz	150	3	36	2
Cherries	7.5 oz	150	2	35	2
Cran-apple juice	8.0 oz	160	—	41	—
Cranberries	11.0 oz	154	1	40	1
Cranberry sauce (unsweetened)	4.0 oz	160	—	44	—
Dates (pitted)	2.0 oz	152	1	42	—
Figs	7.0 oz	147	1	38	1
Fruit (canned/mixed)	1.5 cups	150	3	42	—
Fruit cocktail (unsweetened)	1.5 cups	150	3	42	—
Fruit spread (unsweetened)	6 tbsp	144	—	36	—
Grapes	7.5 oz	150	2	38	2
Grape juice (unsweetened)	9.0 oz	156	2	38	—
Grapefruit	14.0 oz	154	1	38	1

Group IIB cont.

Type	Serving	Calories	P (gm)	C (gm)	F (gm)
Grapefruit juice	12.0 oz	141	1	35	1
Guava	10.0 oz	150	2	34	2
Honey	2.5 tbsp	150	—	40	—
Honeydew melon	15.0 oz	150	2	39	1
Jelly (unsweetened)	3.5 tbsp	158	—	42	—
Kiwi	9.0 oz	153	3	38	1
Lemon	17 oz	145	5	31	—
Lemon juice	2.5 cups	153	2	37	—
Lime	19.0 oz	152	4	34	—
Mandarin orange	12.5 oz	150	3	41	1
Mango	8.0 oz	144	1	38	1
Mulberries	12.5 oz	150	5	35	1
Nectarine	11.0 oz	154	3	36	1
Orange	11.5 oz	150	2	38	1
Orange juice (unsweetened)	12.0 oz	164	—	37	—
Papaya	13.5 oz	149	3	38	1
Papaya nectar	1.0 cup	142	—	36	—
Passion fruit	5.5 oz	149	3	36	—
Peaches	12.5 oz	150	3	39	1
Peaches (canned/ unsweetened)	1.5 cups	150	—	33	—
Pears	9.0 oz	153	1	39	1
Pears (canned/unsweetened)	10.5 oz	150	1	39	—
Persimmons	4.0 oz	144	—	38	—
Pineapple	10.0 oz	154	1	39	1
Pineapple (canned unsweetened)	10.0 oz	150	1	36	—
Pineapple juice (unsweetened)	9.0 oz	150	1	39	—
Plantain	4.5 oz	158	2	41	—
Plums (pitted)	9.0 oz	144	2	33	2
Pomegranate	8.0 oz	152	2	39	1
Prickly pear	12.5 oz	150	3	34	1
Prunes (dried/pitted)	2.0 oz	140	1	36	1
Prune juice (unsweetened)	8.0 oz	160	1	44	—
Raisins	1.75 oz	149	2	39	—
Raspberries	11.0 oz	154	3	36	2
Strawberries	17.0 oz	153	3	34	2
Tangerine	12.5 oz	150	3	40	1
Watermelon	17.0 oz	153	3	34	2

Group IIC
Carbohydrates—Grains, Etc.

Type	Serving	Calories	P (gm)	C (gm)	F (gm)
Bagel (blueberry)	2.0 oz	152	6	30	1
Bagel (cinnamon raisin)	1.75 oz	149	5	29	2
Bagel (egg)	2.0 oz	150	7	29	1
Bagel (garlic)	2.0 oz	160	6	32	1
Bagel (oat bran)	2.25 oz	153	6	32	2
Bagel (onion)	2.0 oz	160	7	31	1
Bagel (plain)	2.0 oz	150	6	30	1
Bagel (poppy seed)	2.0 oz	160	7	29	1
Bagel (pumpernickel)	2.0 oz	160	6	31	1
Beans (baked)	6.0 oz	152	6	33	—
Beans (black, canned)	.75 cup	135	11	32	—
Beans (refried, fat free)	7.5 oz	153	12	32	1
Bread (bran)	1.5 slices	150	6	29	2
Bread (buttermilk)	1.5 slices	150	6	30	2
Bread (corn)	1.5 oz	141	3	22	5
Bread (French)	2.0 oz	156	5	29	2
Bread (granola)	2.5 slices	150	5	30	5
Bread (King's Hawaiian)	1.5 oz	135	5	23	3
Bread (oat bran)	1.25 slices	144	5	24	3
Bread (oatmeal)	2.0 slices	140	4	24	2
Bread (pita, white)	2.0 oz	156	5	32	1
Bread (pita, whole wheat)	2.0 oz	150	6	31	1
Bread (pumpernickel)	2.0 slices	160	6	30	2
Bread (raisin)	1.5 slices	135	3	24	3
Bread (rye)	2.0 slices	140	6	26	2
Bread (7-grain)	1.5 slices	135	4	27	2
Bread (sourdough)	2 slices	130	5	27	1
Bread (white)	2 slices	140	6	26	2
Bread (whole wheat)	3 slices	144	7	30	2
Bun (hamburger, white)	1.25 buns	154	5	27	3
Bun (hamburger, whole grain)	1.0 buns	130	4	20	3
Bun (hot dog, white)	1.25 buns	154	5	27	3
Bun (hot dog, whole grain)	1.25 buns	150	5	24	4
Cereal (bran flakes)	1.5 oz	135	5	33	—
Cereal (oat "O"s)	1.5 oz	167	6	29	3
Cereal (corn flakes)	1.5 oz	165	3	37	—
Cereal (corn grits)	1.5 oz	150	5	33	—
Cereal (creamed rice)	1.5 oz	150	5	33	—
Cereal (creamed wheat)	1.5 oz	150	5	33	—
Cereal (granola, fat free)	1.5 oz	135	3	32	—

Group IIC cont.

Type	Serving	Calories	P (gm)	C (gm)	F (gm)
Cereal (Grape-Nuts)	1.5 oz	150	6	32	—
Cereal (Grape-Nuts Flakes)	1.5 oz	153	5	35	—
Cereal (Malt-o-Meal)	1.5 oz	150	6	32	—
Cereal (oatmeal, unsweetened)	1.5 oz	150	6	29	3
Cereal (puffed corn)	1.5 oz	150	9	33	—
Cereal (puffed rice)	1.5 oz	150	3	36	—
Cereal (puffed wheat)	1.5 oz	150	6	33	—
Cereal (raisin bran)	1.5 oz	130	3	33	1
Cereal (spoon-size shredded wheat)	1.5 oz	150	5	34	1
Cereal (wheat flakes)	1.5 oz	150	4	34	1
Chili (vegetarian, fat free)	10 oz	140	4	23	—
Chips (tortilla, baked)	1.5 oz	165	5	33	3
Corn (canned)	¾ cup	120	3	30	—
Corn (frozen)	¾ cup	120	3	27	—
Corn (raw)	6 oz	144	6	33	3
Crackers (wheat)	1.5 oz	150	3	33	—
Dip (black bean, fat free)	6.5 oz	150	7	26	—
French toast (frozen)	3.0 oz	166	7	27	4
Muffin, English (plain)	1.25 muffins	163	5	32	2
Muffin, English (oat bran)	1.25 muffins	145	5	33	2
Muffin, English (sourdough)	1.0 muffin	135	4	27	1
Pancake (buttermilk frozen)	2.5 oz	150	5	30	2
Pasta (cooked)	4.0 oz	148	5	32	2
Pasta (plain, uncooked)	1.5 oz	150	5	32	2
Pasta (whole wheat, uncooked)	1.5 oz	150	5	32	2
Popcorn (air, unpopped)	1.5 oz	150	5	30	3
Potato (baked)	5.0 oz	150	4	35	—
Potato (sweet)	5.0 oz	150	4	35	—
Pretzels (hard)	1.5 oz	167	4	34	2
Rice (steamed)	.75 cup	150	3	33	—
Rice (brown, uncooked)	1.0 oz	150	3	33	—
Rice (white, uncooked)	1.0 oz	150	3	33	—
Rice cake (honey nut)	1.25 oz	150	3	28	1
Rice cake (plain)	4.0 cakes	140	2	32	1
Snack bar (date)	1 bar	140	3	33	—
Snack bar (raisin)	1 bar	140	3	33	—
Tortillas (corn)	3.0 tortillas	150	3	27	3
Tortillas (flour)	2.0 tortillas	140	4	32	2
Waffles (frozen)	1.0 waffle	130	3	18	5
Yams	5.0 oz	150	4	35	—

Group III
Fat

Type	Serving	Calories	P (gm)	C (gm)	F (gm)
Almond butter (natural)	3 tbsp	255	17	12	21
Almonds (dry roasted)	1.5 oz	255	9	9	23
Avocado	5.0 oz	250	3	10	23
Butter	2.5 tbsp	263	—	—	30
Canola oil	2.0 tbsp	248	—	—	28
Cashew butter (natural)	2.5 tbsp	238	8	10	19
Cashews (dry roasted)	1.5 oz	240	8	14	20
Coconut (raw meat only)	1.0 cup	283	3	12	27
Coconut oil	2.0 tbsp	240	—	—	28
Corn oil	2.0 tbsp	240	—	—	28
Cottonseed oil	2.0 tbsp	240	—	—	28
Cream (half/half)	¾ cup	236	5	8	21
Flaxseed oil	2.0 tbsp	240	—	—	28
Grapeseed oil	2.0 tbsp	240	—	—	28
Guacamole	6.0 tbsp	240	3	3	24
Hazelnut (dry roasted)	1.25 oz	235	4	6	24
Hazelnut butter (natural)	1.25 oz	235	5	6	24
Linseed oil	2.0 tbsp	240	—	—	28
Macadamia butter (natural)	2.5 tbsp	250	3	8	24
Macadamia nuts (dry roasted)	1.25 oz	250	3	5	26
Mayonnaise	2.5 tbsp	250	—	—	28
Mixed nuts (dry roasted)	1.5 oz	240	8	11	21
Olives (pitted)	7.0 oz	259	2	5	27
Olive oil	2.0 tbsp	240	—	—	28
Palm oil	2.0 tbsp	240	—	—	28
Peanut butter (natural)	2.5 tbsp	250	11	8	20
Peanut oil	2.0 tbsp	240	—	—	28
Peanuts (dry roasted)	1.5 oz	255	11	8	23
Peanuts (honey roasted)	1.5 oz	255	11	11	20
Pecans (dry roasted)	1.25 oz	234	3	8	23
Pistachio (dry roasted)	1.5 oz	245	9	11	21
Pistachio butter (natural)	3.0 tbsp	255	9	11	20
Poppyseed oil	2.0 tbsp	240	—	—	28
Rice bran oil	2.0 tbsp	240	—	—	28
Safflower oil	2.0 tbsp	240	—	—	28
Salad dressing (Caesar)	3.5 tbsp	245	4	7	25
Salad dressing (French)	4.0 tbsp	240	—	8	24
Salad dressing (Italian)	4.0 tbsp	240	—	4	24
Salad dressing (ranch)	3.0 tbsp	240	—	3	24

Group III cont.

Type	Serving	Calories	P (gm)	C (gm)	F (gm)
Salad dressing (Russian)	4.0 tbsp	240	—	16	20
Salad dressing (blue cheese)	4.0 tbsp	240	4	8	24
Salad dressing (oil & vinegar)	3.5 tbsp	245	—	4	28
Salad dressing (Thousand Island)	4.0 tbsp	240	—	8	20
Sesame butter	1.5 oz	252	8	9	23
Sesame oil	2.0 tbsp	240	—	—	28
Soybean oil	2.0 tbsp	240	—	—	28
Sunflower oil	2.0 tbsp	240	—	—	28
Sunflower seeds (dry roasted)	1.5 oz	248	8	10	21
Trail mix (nuts, berries)	6.0 tbsp	240	8	32	12
Vegetable oil	2.0 tbsp	240	—	—	28
Walnut oil	2.0 tbsp	240	—	—	28
Walnuts	1.5 oz	270	11	5	26

Group IV

Fast Foods

Arby's

Type	Serving	Calories	P (gm)	C (gm)	F (gm)
Chicken sandwich (grilled barbecue)	1.0 serv.	386	23	47	13
Chicken sandwich (light roast deluxe)	1.0 serv.	276	24	33	7
Roast beef (light deluxe)	1.0 serv.	294	18	33	10
Salad (roast chicken)	1.0 serv.	204	24	12	7

Burger King

Garden salad (no dressing)	1.0 serv.	95	6	8	5
Salad (chunky chicken w/o dressing)	1.0 serv.	142	20	8	4

Carl's Jr.

Charbroiled chicken sandwich	1.0 serv.	310	25	34	6
Roast beef sandwich (roast beef & Swiss)	1.0 serv.	360	31	43	8

continued

Group IV cont.

Type	Serving	Calories	P (gm)	C (gm)	F (gm)
Salad to go (12 oz chicken)	1.0 serv.	200	24	8	8
Teriyaki chicken sandwich	1.0 serv.	330	28	42	6

El Pollo Loco

Chicken breast	3.0 oz	160	26	—	6
Chicken salad (flame broiled)	12.0	160	22	11	4

Hardee's

Chicken breast sandwich (grilled)	1.0 serv.	310	24	39	9
Chicken salad (grilled)	1.0 serv.	120	18	2	4
Chicken salad & pasta	1.0 serv.	230	27	23	3

Jack-in-the-Box

Beef Teriyaki Bowl	1.0 serv.	640	28	124	3
Chicken Teriyaki Bowl	1.0 serv.	580	28	115	2
Chicken Fajita Pita	1.0 serv.	292	24	29	8

KFC

Chicken (rotisserie gold, no skin)	1.0 serv.	199	37	—	6

Long John Silver's

Chicken (lite herb)	1.0 serv.	120	22	1	4
Fish (baked w/ sauce)	1.0 serv.	151	33	—	2
Fish (lemon crumb)	1.0 serv.	150	29	4	1
Fish (lite paprika)	1.0 serv.	120	28	—	—
Fish (scampi sauce)	1.0 serv.	170	28	2	5
Fish entrée (lemon crumb)	1.0 serv.	290	24	40	5
Fish entrée (lite paprika)	1.0 serv.	300	24	45	2
Salad (ocean chef no dressing)	1.0 serv.	110	12	13	1
Salad (seafood)	1.0 serv.	210	14	26	5
Salad (seafood w/ crackers)	1.0 serv.	270	16	36	7
Salad (shrimp w/ crackers)	1.0 serv.	183	27	12	3
Salad (small plain)	1.0 serv.	8	—	2	—

Group IV cont.

McDonald's

Type	Serving	Calories	P (gm)	C (gm)	F (gm)
Milkshake (low-fat chocolate)	10.0 oz	320	11	66	2
Milkshake (low-fat strawberry)	10.0 oz	320	11	67	1
Milkshake (low-fat vanilla)	10.0 oz	290	11	60	1
Salad (chunky chicken)	1.0 serv.	150	25	7	4

Roy Rogers

Chicken breast/wing (no skin)	1.0 serv.	190	32	2	6
Chicken salad grilled	1.0 serv.	120	18	2	4

Shoney's

Charbroiled chicken entrée	1.0 serv.	239	39	1	7
Combo entrée (steak/chicken)	1.0 serv.	239	39	1	7
Fish baked (light side)	1.0 serv.	170	35	2	1
Shrimp (charbroiled)	1.0 serv.	138	25	3	3
Shrimp entrée (boiled)	1.0 serv.	93	20	—	1

Sizzler

Chicken breast	1.0 serv.	151	27	2	4
Cottage cheese (low fat)	1.0 serv.	100	14	4	2
Crab, imitation	1.0 serv.	104	12	14	—
Crab, snow (legs/claws)	1.0 serv.	91	21	—	1
Halibut steak (dinner portion)	1.0 serv.	240	48	—	3
Halibut steak (lunch portion)	1.0 serv.	180	36	—	2
Pollack, breaded	1.0 serv.	140	14	18	1
Salmon (dinner portion)	1.0 serv.	247	32	—	12
Salmon (lunch portion)	1.0 serv.	125	20	—	5
Scallop (breaded)	1.0 serv.	160	14	24	1
Shrimp (broiled)	1.0 serv.	150	23	—	6
Shrimp (scampi)	1.0 serv.	143	27	—	3
Swordfish	1.0 serv.	315	45	—	14
Tuna	1.0 serv.	125	15	—	4

Wendy's

Grilled chicken salad	1.0 serv.	200	25	9	8

About the Author

Cathy Sassin is the Director of the Intrafitt Performance Nutrition and Exercise Center at Gold's Gym, Venice, California. A nationally recognized expert on health and fitness, Sassin has shared her expertise on talk shows such as the *Maury Povich Show*, the *Carol and Marilyn Show*, and *Exhale*, with Candice Bergen; the American Health Network, Discovery Channel, and ESPN; and in magazines such as *Elle*, *Shape*, *Conde Nast Women's Sports and Fitness*, *Men's Fitness*, *Maxim*, *Prime Health and Fitness*, and *Fit Magazine* as well as *Muscular Development*, *Muscle Media*, *Oxygen*, and many more.

One of the world's most accomplished adventure racers, Cathy Sassin has consistently placed in the top three in the Eco Challenge, the Raid Gauloises, the Elf, and the Southern Traverse, the most grueling survival races known. Exhibiting the extreme athletic endurance, skill, and courage needed to cover each four-hundred-mile course on mountain bikes, over glaciers, through jungles and caves, down raging rivers, and across deserts spanning the globe, Cathy is a living testimony of the Gold's Gym way of life.

Over the past two decades, Sassin has counseled, educated, and provided individualized programs for clients ranging from professional athletes and celebrities to those who simply want to look and feel their best. She has helped thousands to have the bodies they always wanted and achieve the performance they had only dreamed about.